Safer Sex
The New Morality

Also by Evelyn Lerman:

Teen Moms: The Pain and the Promise

Safer Sex

The New Morality

By Evelyn Lerman

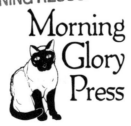

Morning
Glory
Press

Buena Park, California

Library of Congress Cataloging-in-Publication Data
Lerman, Evelyn, 1925-
    Safer sex : the new morality / by Evelyn Lerman.
        p. cm.
    Includes bibliographical references and index.
    ISBN 1-885356-65-X (hc.) – ISBN 1-885356-66-8 (pbk.)
    1. Teenagers—United States—Sexual behavior.
    2. Teenagers—Health and hygiene—United States.
    3. Safe sex in AIDS prevention—United States.
    4. Sexually transmitted diseases—United States—Prevention.
    5. Sexual ethics for teenagers—United States. I. Title.

                            HQ35 .L52 2000
                            306.7'0835—dc21
                            00-035130

            MORNING GLORY PRESS, INC.
    6595 San Haroldo Way   Buena Park, CA 90620-3748
        714/828-1998, 1-888/612-8254   FAX 714/828-2049
                    e-mail mgpress@aol.com
            Web Site http://www.morningglorypress.com
        Printed and bound in the United States of America

CONTENTS

Society has failed our young people. We have given them mixed messages. We have failed to give them the tools to protect themselves. Our statistics on unwanted pregnancy, sexually transmitted disease, and abortion reveal the scope of our failure.

Yet there are places in the world that have found a way to reach and teach their teens about sexual responsibility. As I compared statistics from other developed countries with ours, I resolved to learn the causes of these tremendous differences. To help me find some answers, I participated in a study tour sponsored by Advocates for Youth, Washington, DC, and the University of North Carolina, Charlotte, in the summer of 1998.

In our two weeks in the Netherlands, France, and Germany we learned how these cultures changed from the traditional mores of the forties to their liberal mores of the nineties. We also discovered strong, built-in controls to assure that the greater sexual freedom encompassed the values of respect and responsibility. The goals of their new morality were that all citizens, not only teens, value their own health and safety as well as that of their partners. To achieve these goals, they stressed the importance of practicing safer sex at all times, dramatically lowering the need for abortion, and never knowingly bringing an unwanted child into the world. How did they do it?

By redefining sex as part of the human condition, and by removing the judgmental factor, they said in essence, "People are sexual beings. They will have sex, even if unmarried, and it's our job to help them protect themselves from having abortions. We don't like abortion, even though we acknowledge a woman's right to have one. We will do everything we can to eliminate the need for abortion. It's also our job to protect people from having unwanted children and from getting or giving sexually transmitted diseases."

They told us through discussion, lecture, and interview, and they showed us through the media. We saw true prevention, meaningful prevention, prevention which was where it belonged, in the hands of sexually active people, both adult and teen.

They had come so far with their educational campaigns for safer sex that adults didn't need to impose their will on young people. Adults give youth the message that sexual relationships require responsibility, and young people are able to monitor their own behavior. A teen I interviewed told me that if a young person got pregnant and told a friend, the friend would say, "What's the matter with you? You didn't have to get pregnant. You must be stupid."

And intervention services for teen parents? We neither saw them nor heard about them because there are so few teen parents and so few babies born to teen mothers that there is little need for public programs to care for them. Prevention becomes true intervention. The energy and resources of the government, the schools, the media, the non-governmental agencies, and the parents are focused on safer sex, *the new morality.*

"In the Netherlands, Germany, and France, sexual development in adolescents is seen as a normal and healthy biological, social, emotional, and cultural process," according to tour leaders Linda Berne and Barbara Huberman. "Education focuses on informed choice and sexual responsibility for all members of the society, including adolescents. Public campaigns coordinate with school sexuality education, condom and contraceptive access, and nonjudgmental attitudes from adults to protect sexual health. Scientific research drives sexuality-related public policies in all three nations."

These strategies of prevention are working so well that in the Netherlands only four teens per 1000 give birth each year. The United States' annual rate of *51 births* per 1000 teens is thirteen times as high!

It works in the Netherlands, but many Americans are so consumed with conflicts over teenage sex that they have little energy left to fight the real battle. The real battle is for the protection of teens from pregnancy, abortion, too-early parent-hood, and sexually transmitted infections. The ideological conflict expresses itself through the weapons of the Information Age — words on the internet, newspapers, magazines, music, bulletin boards, billboards, books, pamphlets, and brochures. It continues on the floors of Congress, radio and TV talk shows, speeches in school board meetings, sermons in houses of worship, and in sexuality education classes.

Sometimes the conflict is not in words, but in deeds such as making condoms available in school clinics or bombings and shootings in family planning clinics. Have any gains been made in spite of this conflict? Some might say yes, we have seen gains in a lower birth rate among teens in the past few years. If we look at these "gains" compared with the statistics in the Nether-lands, France and Germany, however, we realize we may have won a skirmish, but we clearly have not won the real battle.

With so many caring people expending so much of their energy, money, time, and effort, how can it be that greater progress is not being made to protect our teens? Is it because we are focusing on the people as adversaries, and not on the prob-lems? Imagine what could happen if all of us who care about teen welfare agreed to pull in one direction? What if we pooled our resources, and decided to attack the real enemies — teen pregnancy, unwanted and unplanned children, unnecessary abortion, sexually transmitted diseases, and teen ignorance about conception and contraception? At the same time we need to work toward eradication of teen illness, teen illiteracy, poverty, sexual abuse, teen hopelessness, teen loneliness, teen vulnerability, and media exploitation. If we agreed to throw teens a safety net encompassing all these things, what could this combined force not accomplish? The thought is heart-stopping.

In which direction could we move? Could those who believe sexual intercourse is right only within marriage and those who appear to advocate sex without responsibility, as so often shown in the media, move toward a middle ground? Could this deep chasm of conflict over teen sexuality be bridged by people on both sides working together for our youth?

This book proposes a new direction entirely, one based on the European model. It is a model that has produced effective results not only for teens, but for the community as a whole. This book will advocate, not for intervention services which we are now providing with some success, but for prevention, that surely is the best intervention.

Safer Sex deals with the history and sociology of teen sexual behavior and the forces which seek to control it. It will explore:
- Sexuality education/abstinence education.
- The role of religion.
- The role of the media.
- Parents as sexuality educators.
- Contraception, including abstinence.
- Abortion.
- AIDS and other sexually transmitted infections.
- Condoms in schools and other accessible locations.
- Effective strategies for preventing teen pregnancy and STIs.

Safer Sex will compare our policies with those of Europe. Finally, it will make recommendations promoting a new morality based on sexual respect, responsibility, and rights on the part of teens as well as on the part of the adults who must set the example for them.

Evelyn Lerman   *June 2000*

For those of us who have been in the field of teen pregnancy prevention for years, there have been times we felt tired and burned out. We wondered if we were ever going to make significant differences in the rates of pregnancy, birth, and sexually transmitted infections in our youth. The good news is that at last the pregnancy and birth rates are declining. Over 80 percent of this reduction is attributed to better and more use of contraception by teens, and 20 percent to teens who are delaying the initiation of intercourse. The bad news is that STI rates, including HIV, continue to escalate. This means our youth may be protecting themselves against pregnancy at times, but not from STIs.

Abstinence until marriage is not a value practiced in this country — over 90 percent of first-time marriages are not virginal. We know most teens become sexually active after 16, and two-thirds of our teen pregnancies occur to 18- and 19-year-olds.

Our youth are observing a sexual and social revolution. The media continue to use sex as the ultimate strategy to lure readers, viewers, and customers. Public figures challenge conventions and become parents without bothering with marriage. Technology in family planning methods gives women the opportunity to engage in intimate sexual relationships without fear of pregnancy. Abortion was legalized as an option for a woman if she did have an unwanted pregnancy.

If over 90 percent of marriages in this country are not virginal marriages, how did the United States allow a small but vocal minority to influence public policy mandating abstinence until marriage for many federal-funded youth programs? Why did they dictate at the local, state and federal level that "abstinence until marriage" is the expected standard for our society? As the age of puberty drops to 11 1/2, and the age of marriage steadily increases (27 in the year 2000), what wisdom prevails to demand that shame, fear, guilt, and inaccurate information will be used to "protect "a young person for well over 15 years from pregnancy and STIs?

Is it not *immoral* to deny young people the information, skills, and services they need to become responsible, respectful sexual human beings? Is it not *immoral* to place their lives in jeopardy because they choose to have intimate sexual relations and don't know what they need to protect themselves and their partners? Is it not *immoral* of our society — our government — to value ignorance and fear-based tactics and to promote guilt and shame in order to try to control behavior? Is it not *immoral* to disenfranchise and disempower young people who *could* and *would* make wise and responsible decisions about sex because *we* are uncomfortable or see only our point of view?

Evelyn Lerman, a participant in the first annual European Study Tour sponsored by Advocates for Youth and the University of North Carolina at Charlotte, offers as a new vision, *Safer Sex: The New Morality.*

With thoughtfulness and courage she has used the study tour experience to help us look at adolescent sexuality in a new way – a way that respects and values young people, supports their *right* to accurate, balanced sexuality education and reproductive health services, and provides youth with the information, skills, and values needed to behave *responsibly.*

As an author and observer who has had an incredible journey throughout her career working with teens and writing about teen parents, she gives us a clear and poignant picture of generations, past and present, and how pregnancy and childbearing affect families, society, and teens themselves. Her words provide us with a picture of what the future will look like — providing we embrace societal, cultural, and public health policies and practices that have led to such incredibly lower rates of teen pregnancy, STIs, and abortion in Western Europe.

Evelyn's insight and ability to reflect on the decades past and to see a vision for the future offers us hope that America can give up the impractical and unhealthy way we address adolescent sexual health.

There are many challenges in this book. For some, these will be eye opening, soul-searching moments. There will be times when Evelyn's boldness and concrete strategies will create discomfort or questions that will be difficult to resolve.

Ultimately though, the reader will leave this book knowing that we *can* have the same results as Western Europe — this rich and diverse America that values individuality and self determination — *if* we have the will and become advocates who stand firm for what we know is right and *moral* for our young people.

Evelyn Lerman has indeed given us a guidebook for the new morality — *Safer Sex or No Sex.*

Barbara Huberman, Training Director
Advocates for Youth, Washington, DC

EDITOR'S COMMENT

For sixteen years I coordinated and taught a teen parent program in Los Angeles County. I saw the trauma experienced by teenagers straddling the two very different worlds of adolescence and parenthood. All loved their children, but many agreed that waiting until they were "ready" to parent would have been far wiser.

Evelyn Lerman and I were roommates on the 1998 teen pregnancy prevention study tour to the Netherlands, France, and Germany. These countries have developed policies that have greatly reduced their teen pregnancy rates. Each also has far lower teen abortion and sexually transmitted infection rates.

We in the United States have a strange attitude toward our youth. We surround them with sex in the media, a fantasy world of sex with no responsibility attached. Pair this with the federal government-funded Abstinence Only programs for youth, another fantasy since half of the 17-year-olds in the U.S. are already sexually active. (The average age for marriage today is 27.) It's a schizophrenic world we offer adolescents.

In the Netherlands, the average age for initiation of sexual intercourse is 17.7 years, almost 11/2 years *later* than in the United States. *Safer Sex: The New Morality* shows the way to help our youth accept their sexuality in a caring, responsible manner.

After many years of writing and publishing books for and about teen parents, I am delighted to be the editor of *Safer Sex: The New Morality.* I truly believe this book can guide us to a better world for our youth.

Jeanne Lindsay, Editor
Author: *Teens Parenting Series*
Teen Dads: Rights, Responsibilities and Joys
Do I Have a Daddy?
Pregnant? Adoption Is an Option
Teenage Couples Series
Books, Babies and School-Age Parents

*Ed. note: We sent manuscripts of **Safer Sex: The New Morality** to a wide variety of people concerned about the high rates of teen pregnancy, sexually transmitted infections including HIV/ AIDS, and abortion in the United States. Many respondents gave us permission to share their comments.*

Jany Rademakers, Netherlands Institute
for Social Sexological Research, The Netherlands:

The discussion about adolescent sexual health policy is extremely polarized most of the time, especially in the USA. People are divided – the "Abstinence only" camp and the "Permissive" camp. Communication between the camps seems impossible, since they adhere only to their own beliefs.

Evelyn has taken the discussion to a higher level. Not only does she try to get at the heart of the people in these camps and provide more understanding of their motivation, but she also tries to base the discussion on evidence instead of beliefs.

What's important to me is that she doesn't portray the European approach as immoral, but that she stresses that norms and values are an essential basis for our policy. Respect and responsibility are key issues in our approach, as well as the right to self-determination.

Henry Rosovsky, Geyser University Professor Emeritus and former Dean of the Faculty of Arts and Sciences, Harvard University:

Evelyn Lerman has an uncanny ability to write about serious and sensitive subjects in a comprehensible, direct, and informative manner. *Safer Sex* will be of great use to parents, teachers, policy-makers — indeed, to all concerned with our future.

Susan N. Wilson
The Network for Family Life Education, NJ:

With *Safer Sex: The New Morality,* Evelyn Lerman has issued a thoughtful, intelligent manifesto for all of us which, if followed, could begin a new era of progress and change in our attitudes about adolescent sexuality and school-based sexuality education programs. For too many years, we have been adopting and implementing public policies, based more on ideology than fact, which do not benefit the majority of our young people. Lerman's book could make a huge difference for children, adolescents, and their families; her approach to these difficult, but crucially important subjects is sensible, clear-eyed and moderate. She deserves our gratitude for showing us a new path.

Marilyn Sanders, School Age Parent Program Coordinator, Lewisville Independent School District, Lewisville, TX:

Our school district recently formed a community-based committee to formulate a K-12 sexuality education curriculum. *Safer Sex: The New Morality* is the perfect book for all committee members to read in order to have a "real picture." It will surely assist in the decision-making that will be critical in developing and implementing a relevant program for our students. It addresses all the pertinent topics and provides current statistics. You have done the homework for us. The insightful *Safer Sex: The New Morality* is exactly what we are experiencing in our work each day with schoolage pregnant and parenting students. Thanks for the opportunity to preview this book!

Lois Gatchell, Deacon, Episcopal Church, Tulsa, OK:

If we truly value the health and safety of our children, we must increasingly bring the volatile sexuality issues into our public forums. Lerman's thoughtful, fact-filled book offers incentive for a new level of dialogue among our health, education, social and religious agencies.

Tom Klaus, Legacy Resource Group, Carlisle, IA:

Safer Sex: The New Morality is very readable and does a nice job of communicating some rather tough issues. . . a valuable book for practitioners, policy makers, parents, and anyone else concerned for the health and well-being of adolescents.

Carol Cassell, Centers for Disease Control and Prevention, Atlanta, GA:

Safer Sex: The New Morality is a splendid, landmark book with the power of a revelation. It is a rich and informative account of why our nation has such appallingly high rates of adolescent pregnancy and childbearing compared to other western industrialized countries. Evelyn Lerman clearly reframes issues that have been endlessly debated for decades. She offers imaginative solutions not only rooted in research, but in common sense guided by a moral commitment to young people. This is essential reading for everyone in public policy, health and social services, and especially those who are sincerely interested in the prevention of adolescent pregnancy. I highly recommend it.

Rev. Anita Iceman, Orangethorpe United Methodist Church, Fullerton, CA:

It's a terrific book, a wonderful approach. I think a lot of people will respond positively.

Linda Miklowitz, Attorney, Tallahassee, FL:

As a mother of two teenagers, a NOW chapter president, and a former journalist turned lawyer, I am impressed by Evelyn Lerman's clear writing and clear thinking about the explosive issue of sexual relations and young people. She offers not only a lucid description of the problem, but also good suggestions for helping young people.

Michael McGee, Vice President for Education, Planned Parenthood Federation of America, Inc., New York, NY:

Lerman has done an admirable job of articulating the argument for a more rational and pragmatic approach to adolescent sexual behavior.

The Rev. Dr. Marilynn Huntington, Director, Council on Ministries, California Pacific Annual Conference of the United Methodist Church:

This is an honest, comprehensive look at an enormous problem in our society. It is carefully and thoroughly researched. The book clearly makes a case for a new look at sex education in America. The "European" model is unheard of here — largely due to a fundamentalist mentality. Though it is undoubtedly true, I grieve that it is the "church" that is the roadblock to a healthier attitude toward sex education.

Genie Wheeler, MSW, columnist, retired social worker:

The theme of this remarkable book is "attack problems, not people." The author not only advocates this approach but demonstrates how it can be implemented by the way she writes. On the volatile, emotional issues of abortion, contraception, and sexuality education Ms. Lerman is non-judgmental as she describes different points of view with empathy and respect.

Then she goes beyond that to find common values and common goals. She covers all aspects, comparing U.S. policies with those of other developed countries. *Safer Sex* . . . is well-researched, comprehensive, and compelling.

If *Safer Sex* could be required reading for school board members, congressmen, parents, and all who have strong feelings about these issues, teen pregnancy, AIDS, STIs, etc., would be considered health issues based on scientific principles rather than political and wildly controversial polarizing challenges.

Ms. Lerman is not only scientifically oriented, but a philosopher and an ethicist. Her book is a wonderful blend of interviews, the human touch, hard scientific research, and advice and experience of the author. It's very much a needed book.

Catherine A. Sanderson, Department of Psychology, Amherst College, Amherst, MA:

The book is compelling on many levels — very readable, nice blend of facts and statistics plus personal interviews and anecdotes. Provides a new and insightful perspective on many issues. I can see it being used successfully by parents and educators.

Rabbi Allan H. Schwartzman, Sarasota, FL:

Evelyn Lerman's *Safer Sex: The New Morality* is an eye-opener for every one of us. Fathers and mothers (grandparents too), teens, teachers, clergy, and elected officials need to read and learn. All of us can do better; all of us *must* do better in this crucial and controversial area of living in America in the new century. Evelyn Lerman has made a profound and necessary contribution to our thinking. She has backed it by practical research. Now, it is for us to read and react.

Sharon Morrill, Health Educator, Newcastle, ME:

Evelyn Lerman's first book, *Teen Moms: The Pain and the Promise,* shifted my paradigm regarding teen pregnancy. She has taken an even more courageous step in *Safer Sex*, a valuable read for anyone who works with, lives with, cares for or educates teens.

Rev. Douglas W. Drown, Bingham, ME:

Safer Sex is well-documented, well-thought out, and incisive.

Joyce Delgado, Independent Study Teacher, Redding, CA:

What a novel concept this book conveys — to teach our children about a natural bodily function, sexuality, with knowledge and compassion.

One of the goals of *Safer Sex: The New Morality* is to have all adults and their agencies work together to educate our youth about abstinence, conception, and contraception — all the methods that would prevent abortions, unwanted children, unplanned pregnancies and STIs.

No matter what morals adults foster — I don't care — what concerns me is the immorality, or dare I say stupidity, of losing our children to preventable at-risk behaviors.

Rev. George Pasley, United Presbyterian Church, Garnett, KS:

I like the pragmatism of *Safer Sex: The New Morality*. It does not leave out the option of abstinence, but recognizes its difficulty. I hope those of us who recognize abstinence as a moral issue can provide guidance that is not based on fear and shame, but on positive reasons. This book can help us.

Judy Glynn, RN, Chairperson, Rural Northeast Kansas AIDS Task Force:

When I was growing up, sex was not discussed or taught, only the rule, "No sex." Many parents today recognize that is not enough and worry, not just about their children getting pregnant but dying from AIDS. Just saying "No sex" never was enough nor was it a healthy approach to embracing the gift of human sexuality. The facts in Evelyn Lerman's book speak for themselves.

How do we break that cycle? It can only be through education and information, not to abandon our own values and morality but to expand them. *Safer Sex: the New Morality* recognizes that abstinence still is the best choice, but addresses the fact that many people, young and old, do not make that choice. This book does not abandon them to the consequences, but provides us not only with factual information, but the opportunity to hear from many different points of view. Then we have a challenge: to work together to create a comprehensive approach to the issues of human sexuality and the consequences of our choices. In today's world, both for the unborn and the living, it's a matter of life and death.

Jean Brunelli, PHN, La Palma, CA:

Safer Sex: The New Morality is a treatise on the shifting paradigm for the health, social service, and education systems of the country. It puts forth thoughtful discussion and concrete suggestions. Reading this book would give teachers an opportunity to pull back and reflect on what they're doing and how it fits into the scheme of things. It would be good for school board members and for people in all the helping services who have concerns about teen pregnancy.

Linda Berne, Professor,
University of North Carolina, Charlotte:

Finally, someone with the guts to write a book that tells the whole truth!

Pam Kinnan, TeenAge Pregnancy/Parenting Facilitator,
North Heights Alternative School, Amarillo, TX:

Evelyn Lerman has written a book that contains all that I believe about the prevention of unplanned pregnancy, abortion, and sexually transmitted diseases. I say that because I am in complete agreement that we, as a whole society, need to help prevent teen pregnancy, STIs, and abortion through comprehensive sexuality education and accessibility of contraception methods.

The Netherlands, Germany, and France have come to terms with the volatile, value-laden issues of *preventing* teen pregnancy, STIs, and abortion. Isn't it time that we as a nation resolve our differences of conflicting values regarding teenage sex, unmarried sex, contraception and abortion in order to benefit our young people? *Safer Sex: The New Morality* is a book that can show us the way. For those of us who advocate for youth, this book should be required reading.

Rev. Jim Brewster, United Methodist Church,
Rowland Heights, CA:

I especially liked the theory behind the book. The author did an excellent job of giving the reader a *sound* understanding of why the A+ (teaching about abstinence *and* contraception) is so necessary. I have been an ordained minister in the United Methodist Church for many years, and have heard all of the rhetoric about abstinence only — and feel it is entirely short-sighted and unrealistic. Teen pregnancy and STIs have soared while the religion, media, and politics have maintained their pious views that the only way is abstinence. I agree with the author that while abstinence is the preferable method for adolescents, it is mandatory that everyone *must* have the knowledge that comes with A+ to make a significant difference. I felt that the author made an outstanding contribution in this book to present a workable program which deals with the problems and avoids attacking people. The author makes an important contribution in the precise layout of moving toward the new morality. I applaud her dedication to the task.

Marie Mitchell, RN, Grady Memorial Hospital, Atlanta, GA
Co-author, *Postponing Sexual Involvement:*

Safer Sex provides a simple, logical and common sense approach to addressing the issue of Abstinence Only versus Abstinence Plus. The question was asked, "Are we dreaming to think these two points of view can come to terms with each other for the benefit of our young people?" Probably, but we must continue to be a voice crying in the wilderness and believe that dreams do come true. We can't afford not to.

ACKNOWLEDGMENTS

Thank you to

. . . my friends and family who understood and put up with me when I was not available.

. . . Carole, Karen and Bob at Morning Glory Press for all their help and many kindnesses.

. . . Hannah Honeyman and Linda Miklowitz for their diligence in keeping me informed on the internet.

. . . Barbara Huberman, Linda Berne, Peggy Brick, Sharon Rodine, Tom Klaus, Barbara Levy, Anita Mitchell, Catherine Sanderson, Susan Wilson, Sharon Merrill, Pam Kinnan, Rabbi Allan Schwartzman, Michael McGee, Sara Sellinger, Rev. Frank Hawkins, Rev. Donald Drown, Carol Cassell, Sr. Maureen Joyce, Jean Brunelli, Laurie Zabin, Henry Rosovsky, Genie Wheeler, Tom Klaus, Rev. Marilynn Huntington, Rev. Jim Brewster, Marie Mitchell, Rev. Anita Iceman, Joyce Delgado,

Erin Lindsay, Bobbie Westgate, Judy Glynn, Midge Ransom, Lois Gatchell, Marilyn Sanders, Rev. George Pasley, and the many other pre-publication readers who so willingly and generously shared their expertise.

. . . staff at the Alan Guttmacher Institute, the National Campaign to Prevent Teen Pregnancy, Advocates for Youth, SIECUS, ASHA, the Rhode Island Department of Health, Lorraine Colby and the staff at the Sarasota Cyesis Teen Parent Program, the Network for Family Life Education, Representative Dan Miller, Planned Parenthood in Washington and Sarasota, and the Source Teen Theatre, all of whom answered questions and sent research data promptly and with good grace.

. . . the interviewees in the United States, the Netherlands, France, Switzerland, Italy, England, and Germany for talking with me about their experiences.

. . . Dr. Jany Rademakers who opened her world to us with charm, honesty, and understanding.

. . . and to Jeanne Warren Lindsay — coach, confidante, editor, publisher, friend.

Evelyn Lerman, Sarasota, Florida

To Allie, my dear husband and best friend,
whose unfailing good humor and loving support
made *Safer Sex: The New Morality* possible.

"IF" for parents

If you had a son,
would you want the best for him —
the very best?
I think you would,
I know I would.

And if you had a daughter,
would you wish for her the best —
the very best?
I know you would,
I know I would.

And if the best could not be had,
what would you have for them?
surely not the worst —
not tragedy, not life wasted,
No —
there would be no joy in that.

No, for your children
you would want instead
the best that they could have,
the best that they could do —
honesty, and faithfulness,
and thoughtfulness
Let them learn the joy in that,
and so find in everything
the best that life can be.

© by Rev. George R. Pasley
United Presbyterian Church
Garnett, KS
April 17, 2000

INTRODUCTION

Why does the United States have so much difficulty controlling its rate of teen pregnancy, birth, sexually transmitted diseases and abortion while most western European countries are solving these problems?

- Why do 51 teens out of every thousand give birth each year in the United States while the number drops to 14 per 1000 in Germany, nine per 1000 in France, and an amazing four per 1000 in the Netherlands?

- Why is our abortion rate per thousand teenagers almost six times higher than in the Netherlands?

- Why are teens in the United States much more likely to contract a sexually transmitted infection (STI)?

- Why do our teens initiate sexual intercourse *earlier* than any of these European countries, almost 1 1/2 years earlier than in the Netherlands?

Although both the United States and Europe experienced the Sexual Revolution of the sixties, each developed in different ways after that. Yes, we had the pill and access to abortion just as the Europeans did, but our basic attitudes toward sexuality did not change. In Europe, particularly in the pragmatic Netherlands, people re-examined their attitudes. They decided to be realistic about the fact that teens are sexual human beings just as adults are.

Is there a difference between a society and its culture? In a small fairly homogeneous country like the Netherlands, the society and the culture are much the same. People have no need to defend what is "theirs" because everything is "ours." But in a large, heterogeneous country where many cultures form a loosely constructed society, people are in conflict over whose values, whose lifestyles, whose conventions will prevail.

In *The Culture of Intolerance,* Professor Mark Nathan Cohen defines society as "a group of people who interact with one another"[1] and culture as "the mostly unwritten rules and conventions of thought, communication, and behavior that people use" to interact.

When groups of people have different rules there is bound to be conflict. The extremes in the United States range from "Young people have the right to decide how they will live their sexual lives and adults need take no responsibility for their behavior" to "Only abstinence from sexual intercourse until marriage is the appropriate behavior for young people."

Early in the twentieth century the Melting Pot ethic was an attempt to make everyone into Americans. Much of the society and the culture appeared to mesh as one. Today, with ethnic groups from dozens of countries in every major city, people don't want to "melt," nor are they expected to. In Brookline, Massachusetts, where my family grew up, there are the flags of fifty countries hanging in the high school cafeteria. When we were school children, the town was Caucasian, middle to upper middle class, one flag flying. Today it is multi-ethnic, lower class to upper middle class. The families are Caucasian, African American, Asian, Indian, and Hispanic, with many flags flying.

There used to be only Catholic churches, Protestant churches, and Jewish synagogues. Now there are those plus Buddhist, Muslim, Greek Orthodox, and Hindu houses of worship. Some churches have disappeared altogether, displaced by apartments and condominiums for new residents.

As for political persuasions, when I was a school teacher/ administrator from 1967 to 1992, there was a small right-wing fundamentalist minority in this mostly liberal town. They complained bitterly in the press, at school committee meetings, and in the schools about the "touchy-feely" social studies curric- ulum replacing solid geography and history. They mourned that the literature program was sliding away from traditional English and European authors into vague multiculturalism. They fought sex education and the proposal to put condoms in the nurse's clinic in the high school. But they didn't have much clout.

They have a lot more power today.

"A society can easily be at odds with its own members" says Professor Cohen, which is perhaps an understatement of today's conditions in the United States. As an example he writes, "Our society has imposed all kinds of arbitrary rules that make breastfeeding difficult, such as our culturally defined sexual obsession with breasts and fairly arbitrary standards of decency, which treat breastfeeding in public as if it were indecent expo- sure."[2] Surely this is at odds with some members of our society, the women who have to carry their babies with them as they go to work, to shop, to the doctor, or to visit. Few poor families can afford day care and fewer may know how to express milk into a bottle so the baby can be fed breast milk by someone else. Even fewer have the "someone else."

How is it that in our culture breasts are beautified and criti- cized at the same time? When they are exposed for the benefit of male voyeurism, they are beautiful. When they are utilized to provide milk for babies, they are vilified.

A Personal History of the Twentieth Century

Let's take a look at our history through the eyes of some people who were teens in the United States during the decades spanning the twentieth century. Before each interview, I discussed the lessons I had learned in Europe. I talked about the Netherlands in particular where a mass media campaign of ads teaches "safe sex or no sex." These ads can be seen on TV any hour of the day. I described how schools provide sexuality education from the earliest grades, and how the attitude about teen sex is not judgmental or moralistic. With government funding, the media, the schools, and the clinics provide education, access to contraception, and referral for abortion if needed.

I told the interviewees that, along with their rights, Dutch teens are expected to be respectful and responsible for their own and their partners' health and well-being. They are expected to avoid sexually transmitted infections, abortion, and unwanted, unplanned children through abstinence or other responsible methods of contraception.

After filling them in on my perceptions of the Netherlands, I asked them to tell me what life was like for young people when they were in their teens.

The interviewees ranged in age from 14 to 100.

The 1910s

Nana Jeanne, 100. My mother-in-law for fifty-two years, great-grandmother of 11, Nana Jeanne was 15 in 1912. Born in 1897, she died in 1999, her life spanning almost three centuries. A remarkable woman, Nana Jeanne realized there had been change, and while she loved the idea of opportunity and freedom for women, she thought things had gone too far. What's more, she believed young people thought so, too. She spent her last five years in an assisted living home where she talked with the aides and nurses. These are the young women she talks about here, many of them single parents, who shared with her how difficult life was for them.

First of all you must remember that in my day when I was growing up as a teenager, we didn't know about sex. When the girls got together in a group they said to each other, "Where do babies come from?" I was probably 14 or 15 because I was only 16 when I graduated, and I was a very shy child. I didn't mingle too much with the older girls, but I did listen. They used to say they knew where babies come from — the mother's belly — but who put it there? That was about all the sex we knew. As I grew older, naturally we talked more about it, with the older girls and my cousins who were my age and older, but we didn't know what the actual sex act was about. In those days we really lived a very virginal, quiet girl's life.

Then of course we all went to work and we mingled with men older than ourselves, some nice, some not so nice. We learned to take care of ourselves and let no man manhandle us. Then, when I got married, we knew so little, I wonder how we ever made babies. There was no such thing as foreplay. It was wham, bam, thank you ma'am. I don't think in my day people liked sex, or maybe it was just me, but I didn't enjoy it. It was something I had to do for my husband. I don't think the men were very polished either about what they were doing.

I really don't know why the young teenagers in the late fifties and sixties went so free and wild. It was probably because society brought so much to their attention — sex, pornography, movies — all encouraging them in their desire for freedom. But I think it's on the wane, I really do. Young girls who have babies have a certain responsibility that they are not shirking. They love their babies, but it ties them down so they can't do what they want. I think from now on the generations who've seen all that are going to be more circumspect.

The 1920s

Ula. Born in 1911, Ula is now close to 90. She grew up in an academic community and was privileged to attend college in the days when women rarely did. It was illegal to display contraceptives in pharmacies in Connecticut in the 1920s. She learned about contraception when she spent her junior year in France. Most young ladies didn't partake of sex, she told me, but they knew that certain gentlemen of means had mistresses or visited prostitutes.

We had sex education at home from our mother, but the teachers were too shy to talk about sex in school. I went to my first dance when I was 13. He was my cousin's cousin and he treated me very respectfully. We were too young to drive so our parents transported us, and I never had the opportunity to be alone with a boy in a car. All parties were chaperoned. The first party I ever had at home was when I was twelve. We invited boys, and only one showed up. We girls tore him apart trying to dance with him.

In high school we went to dances and we necked and petted. Necking was rather restrained, and petting was a bit more involved. I know there was plenty of that going on.

In college, we had to sign out and say exactly where we were going. We protected our friends by signing them out for the night and saying they were going to a friend's house. Actually they were in a neighboring town with a boyfriend. I never heard of anyone getting pregnant, and there were no babies.

It wasn't until I got to college that I was offered science. Only the boys had science in high school. Freshman year in college we had Hygiene 101, and that's when we were introduced to our bodies. Most of us were still ignorant about the actual means of reproduction.

*My mother and I were close. She talked to me as young as nine that I should expect to menstruate, but I knew nothing about young men. My brother tells me they gave him a book to read called **What Every Young Man Should Know,** but I had no book. Mother told me nothing about contraception.*

Things were very different then. In 1927 a gynecologist friend of the family got into trouble when he performed an abortion on a woman who later died. He was sent to Sing Sing!

There was a 20-year old girl we knew who had a "eugenic" child. She picked a man to get her pregnant and then had her child. We were all amazed she did that.

We were sexually aware enough to fall in love with Rudolph Valentino.

I remember the first boy I ever fell for. I was twelve, and when he came to my front door, I flipped!

I graduated from Smith at 19, very young, but couldn't go to Yale because women weren't admitted then. At Smith we heard rumors about a group of women who lived in a particular wing in a special dormitory. There were whispers about them so we were aware of homosexuals, of lesbians and gay men.

Even with a college education I never became a career lady on my own. I taught a little, then married my husband. When he became a doctor, I worked side by side with him in the office for 33 years. I ran the office and the business part.

When I was a young woman, even in Europe, there were always chaperones at a party. Now I really don't know. There is no chaperoning. I think teens shouldn't have sex at least until college because they are too immature, too irresponsible, too young to know the consequences.

We need better sex education, we need to teach responsibility. Our whole moral texture is so different today. We are missing something in our whole way of life.

I wouldn't want to provide contraception to the very young, even through clinics. There should be more education, even for the parents, by the schools, the churches and temples, so they'd know how to teach their children. Now they are not watching them, not teaching them. Maybe we don't have to talk too much about morality, but we surely can talk about responsibility.

The 1930s

Aaron. A grandparent interviewed in his mid-eighties, Aaron grew up in the Northeast, the son of immigrant parents, one of four siblings. Life was very simple then, he recalled, and boys were more interested in sports and eating than they were in girls.

I grew up the youngest in a family of two sisters and one brother. Nobody ever talked to me about sex, not at home and not in school. The boys in high school had a tight-knit group and the girls did, too. For some reason or other we decided that we weren't going to have anything to do with them, and we weren't going to date at all.

We went all the way through high school without having anything to do with the girls. We played football and basketball and some sandlot baseball, and we kept very busy. A few of the boys broke the compact, but most of us stayed with it.

It wasn't until college that I really got interested in girls. I don't think most of us had sex until we were in our twenties. As for the girls, all I know is there were a couple of girls that everyone said were "loose," but not many.

A lot of the time we had, in addition to the six of us, between ten and twelve other relatives eating and sleeping at our house. They were the relatives from Europe who my mother and father were bringing over to this country. They lived with us until they could find jobs and make it on their own.

I did take some science courses in college, but no biology. I never really learned anything about the body except through trial and error. But it didn't seem to hurt me or my friends. We all managed to get through our childhoods and young adulthood, go to school, and then to work. I was trained to be an engineer, but there were no jobs then, so I went to work for my father in the construction business. That's where I worked until I retired.

The 1940s

Mary and Clayton. Grandparents, raised in the South, now retired and in their seventies, Mary and Clayton were 15 in 1944. Their dilemma is that they remember their own upbringing in a Southern town when things were still very controlled. They did have to deal with their children in the sixties, and they had to make some changes. But this generation — having babies without being married — is very frightening for them.

Times have really changed. I worked in a drugstore in the late 40s. It was a Catholic stronghold we lived in then. There were no contraceptives in the store. People asked for them, but the owners wouldn't stock them.

I hope my children educate their children more, and at younger ages than we did. We worried when ours were in high school; they have to worry while theirs are in grade school.

We are in a funny position to answer your question about what our children should tell our grandchildren. They adopted a baby who was born to unmarried teen parents. We love that child. It's going to be difficult for the parents to talk with him about premarital sex because he is a product of that.

The 1950s

Natalie. Now in her early sixties. A grandparent and career woman in Maine, Natalie was 15 in 1954. She is a Roman Catholic who talks about her upbringing in parochial schools with humor and love. Natalie had to decide for herself about birth control, a conflict with which many Catholics have had to deal. She raises this question as she asks how the Netherlands' policies could be implemented here.

Well, it (Netherlands system) *certainly sounds reasonable and something that would work in a nation like the Netherlands, but I guess I have more questions than responses. My first question is how would this work in a nation that is as Puritanical as the United States? People say this nation is not Puritanical, but we all know that it is. It's based on the Puritan ethic where sex is a no-no, particularly if you're Roman Catholic like I am.*

I joke with my friend Barbara and say if you're raised Catholic, cards are OK but sex is not, but if you're raised Baptist, sex is OK but cards are not.

In theory, what you told me certainly goes along with my thinking. One of the problems in this country is there is so much emphasis out there on sex, with it hanging out all over. I think it's probably a reaction to this Puritanical thing we all have about sex.

The 1960s

Chuck, 53. A parent, Chuck was 15 in 1962, and describes himself as a political conservative, a social liberal, and a used-to-be Catholic. He tried to live in the way that was best for his family. He raised his children accordingly, making sure his sons knew exactly how to protect themselves and the women with whom they had sexual relationships. You hear his conservative attitudes in his political discussion and his liberal attitudes in his views on family life.

I was brought up in the 60s. I graduated in 1964. Drugs were nothing to us, we hardly knew anything at all about them. As for sex, we were going to parochial school. They advised us definitely to stay away from sex, to practice abstinence (laughing). *There were a lot of taboos associated with it. Not that we didn't try to score, but the girls were not as submissive as they were in later years.*

That's the way things were back then. Condoms were available, but always behind the pharmacy counter. We had to stammer and stumble, and you couldn't call them condoms, you had to call them prophylactics.

It was kind of an uncomfortable situation then, and the worst thing you could do was get a girl pregnant. Things were different then than they are now.

The 1970s

Gracie, 40. A parent of five, a social worker with teen parents, Gracie was 15 in 1974. Educated by a caring teacher, she still worries about what happened to her mentor. That was in the 70s, yet even today we have teachers who are afraid to address the issue of contraception in their sexuality education classes.

I'm certainly for the Dutch method. A lot of people say, "But you're giving them permission to have sex." I don't think we're giving them permission. I think they are deciding for themselves. One way or the other some are going to do it. Teenagers are teenagers, and if we give them the information to be safe, that's better than just having them sneak around and be unsafe. I feel that way because I might have been a teen mother if it hadn't been for a wonderful high school health teacher who taught us about contraception. When the school found out, they fired her. I've tried to find her since, but no one knows where she went.

One of the things I stress with the teen moms I work with is carry condoms with you. Don't rely on anybody else. It's your body. You have to protect yourself. Go into the store and buy them. Sometimes I go on field trips with them and take them to the drugstore and have them buy them.

I took my daughter, too, at 15, and showed her where condoms were, explained about them, and then had her buy them. I hoped that when she became sexually active, she'd be able to buy them without being embarrassed or shy. She didn't become sexually active until she was 18. I just wanted her to be ready.

I did the same thing with my son when he was 16. He was not showing any interest at all in girls. I waited until I saw his face light up when he saw the cheerleaders, and I knew the hormones were starting to flow. I told him it was time to talk, and we talked. Then I took him to the drugstore just like I did with my daughter.

The 1980s

Liz, 26. Born in the United States, Liz's parents divorced when she was young. Her mother raised her in the United States and overseas, and she lived with her dad about 15 percent of the time. We interviewed her when she was living and working in Paris.

*Mom showed me **The Joy of Sex** when I was about nine. She read it with me and we talked about it. I knew enough to protect myself, and I had sex for the first time at 14. My dad found out about it by snooping in my room and reading a note I had written. He made me call my mother, who was 3,000 miles away, to tell her. Even though we were best friends and confidantes, I hadn't told her. Somehow I knew she wouldn't approve.*

When I told her over the phone with my father listening, she told me that what I had done was something I'd always regret. About a year later, when I was 15 years old, she came to grips with it and bought me lacy teddies, reimbursed me for the birth control pills I was taking, and allowed my boyfriend to sleep over with me.

My dad was very matter-of-fact about it, and immediately took me to the doctor to get a prescription for the pill. He never mentioned it again. By the time I was 17, I'd had three lovers. Now in my late twenties, I have had 13. Not necessarily figures I'm proud of, but definitely not a source of shame, or, I dare say, regret.

I think Americans are too repressed about sex. It's natural and should not be taboo. If I have children I'll want them to be safe.

As long as my child has safe sex, I honestly don't care when they
start having sex.

Of course I'm pro-choice and think abortion is a viable option
for some people. The world is overpopulated as it is. I don't
know, but I don't think I would be able to do it myself if I were
with someone for whom I genuinely cared. It totally depends on
maturity and awareness of complications and risks involved. Yet
I thought I was mature enough at 14 when I first had sex.

The 1990s

Lauren, 17. Mother of an 18-month old son. I interviewed
Lauren in a pregnant and parenting teen high school. Her story
follows the pattern of teen mothers having daughters who
become teen mothers. She lives with her baby's father, and he's a
good dad.

Imagine the change in mores from the days of Nana Jeanne,
who didn't know what sexual intercourse was until she got
married. Today Lauren, who worried that her boyfriend might
leave her if she didn't have sex with him, is pleased that he never
pressured her and waited a "whole month and a half" to have
sex. At 15 she has forged a relationship in which they are faithful
to each other. She feels lucky. But what must life have been for
this young woman who at 14 moved in with a 15-year-old?

I asked her to tell me when she began having sex and how it
happened.

When I met my baby's father I was 14, he was 15. He's the
only person I've ever had sex with. He had it before but he
doesn't cheat now.

We've been together for three and a half years and we're both
faithful. I treasure it. He's a very good dad. His name is Richard
and the baby is Richard, Jr. He works as a carpenter, framing
buildings. He wants me to finish high school. He encourages me
and helps me. He can read but not too well, and he may go back
to school. I'm going to get a job so we can move out of my
mother's house.

I had sex with him at 14. He was 15. At first we were together
without having sex. I worried he'd leave me if I didn't have sex

with him, but he waited a whole month and a half. He was being pressured by the guys to have me, but he didn't push me. Then I decided to have sex.

We always used contraception, but this one time it broke. Mom and I are close, and I got the pill recently. Back then I didn't know it was available or I would have taken it.

The doctor gave me foam when my mom wasn't in the room, but he never discussed the pill with me. She never did either. If I'd had more education, I'd never have gotten pregnant. My mother was 16 when she had her first child.

Tina, 15. Mother of a one-year old, Tina attends a high school for pregnant and parenting teens. Tina, who had a baby at 14, found her mentor in a teen mother. That's an irony in itself. She was lucky, too, for this woman who loved her got her off drugs and away from a bad crowd. But she also advised her that having a baby would help her settle down.

Tina followed the advice, then married. Although she is having a good experience in this school for teen parents, she has given up her childhood.

There was a couple that cared a lot about me when I was growing up. The woman had been a teen mother. I loved her and she loved me. She wanted me to go to college, stop smoking, stop doing drugs (weed, Ecstasy), stop drinking, stop shoplifting, get out of the bad crowd I was in. She also made me want to have a baby and a family. She said once I did that I'd stop doing all the wild things and I'd settle down. So I had a baby and now I'm happily married.

I wouldn't change anything except I wish I hadn't done drugs and gone with that bad crowd. Sometimes I feel I'm too young to be a mother, but I don't regret my baby. I don't regret him, but a little later would have been better. I'm waiting to get a house, want to learn the computer, want to be a teacher.

I never had friendships and fun. I slept with guys but it never meant anything. I don't ever want to leave this school. I love it. I've been here for two years.

What is our society saying to these young women? We don't approve of your behavior and we won't help you prevent pregnancy. We can't meet your needs in traditional high schools, but if you get pregnant we'll educate you and your child. What is it saying to Colette who is 15 now, has a five-month-old son, and became sexually active at 13? She told me, "Sex education wouldn't have helped me much. In fact, it didn't help me at all. In the sixth grade I don't remember very much about it except that I had already lost my virginity and I was on my way to sex education class."

What is it saying to Fionia, mother of 16-year old Chad? Chad came to her on the Fourth of July to tell her he'd had sex the night before. They'd run out of condoms, but they took a chance. He was nervous now and wanted his mother to find him the morning after pill (emergency contraception). Although it was legal in their state and she worked in social services, she couldn't locate anyone who would give it to her for her son's teen partner.

Chad's baby was delivered nine months later. By then he was separated from the mother of his child. However, he gave up his plans to go away to college and chose a community college near home so he could spend time with his daughter on the weekends.

We've got it all backwards, don't you think?

1

From Prudery
to Pragmatism

*I'd say to younger kids, stay away from sex if you can,
but if you can't, use protection. I made bad decisions. I
decided to have sex and I didn't protect myself, so here I
am pregnant and about to have a baby. I'm smart and I'm
a good student, but I sure wasn't smart about this.*

Josie, 17, Florida

Picture yourself seated in an auditorium with 1000 average
girls aged 15 to 19 from all over the United States. Here is some
information about them:[1,2]

- Half of the 17-year-olds have had sexual intercourse.
- The median age at which they initiate sexual intercourse is
  16.3 years.
- 125 have a sexually transmitted infection.
- 100 are pregnant.
- 70 of these pregnancies were unintentional.

- About 15 will miscarry.
- 27-30 will have an abortion.
- At least 51 of these young women will become mothers.
- Less than 30 of the 100 pregnant girls are married.

If we truly want to help our children delay sexual intercourse, develop a healthy sexuality, avoid pregnancy and sexually transmitted infections, and reduce abortion, we must change *our* ways. We must work together on these common goals, whether we are deeply religious or not aligned with a religion, whether in our political thinking we lean toward the Left or the Right, and whether our view on the abortion issue is pro-life or pro-choice.

First, we need to look at our culture, at the mores that guide our thinking and our actions.

What have we learned about sexual attitudes and behaviors over the course of this century? What does sex look like in the new millennium? It's not the "making out" of the past. That was our term for kissing, heavy petting, and sexual exploration. Today "making out" means "doing it." "It" means different things to different people. Vaginal sex, oral sex, and anal sex have definitions of their own. Some people subscribe to the notion that unless it's vaginal sex it isn't really sex at all. You're a technical virgin as long as you haven't had vaginal sex. And you're a "secondary virgin" after you've had vaginal sex and then you decide to abstain again.

"Technical virginity" and "secondary virginity" make me think of the Inuit in Alaska, who have more than fifty words for "snow." They need them because snow is such an important part of their lives. They distinguish between the snow that is safe to walk on, to sled on, the snow that will help a hunt, the snow that could crush an igloo, and the snow that could protect the ice. We, who worry only about shoveling the driveway and skidding, don't need as much vocabulary.

Today's sexual mores, being far more complicated than in the past, demand more vocabulary for sex. Movies, magazine covers, music, radio talk shows, and TV programs bare all, including people's deepest feelings and emotions. Because we have gone so far, it takes more and more to get our attention. As a friend says, "Everything is hanging out all over." Women's magazines now include photographs that used to be found only as centerfolds in *Playboy*.

Sex has been demystified and marketed in the same way we package cookies. Even if the cookies don't taste marvelous, the packaging promises that they will. Attraction is all. Young people know this, just as older people do.

Different Views on Nudity

Europeans and Americans don't agree in their attitudes about nudity. In the world of real flesh and blood, Americans are skittish about naked bodies. Two adult males recently told me that they were amazed when they looked down on the beach from a hotel terrace in Sarasota, Florida, and saw two young women sunbathing topless while their children were playing nearby. For these European women, that was the norm and neither they nor their children thought anything of it.

On a trip to Europe this past summer, when our tour group was shown a mineral springs spa in Baden-Baden, Germany, the guide mentioned that all bathing and treatments are done in the nude. The American group I was with looked shocked and uncomfortable. I asked several women if anyone would be interested in going with me, but there were no takers. Yet, for German women, it's the most natural thing in the world.

Massage in Europe also illustrates the difference in attitudes. After an exercise session in the pool, I entered the massage room where a masseur greeted me. When he asked me to disrobe I told him I was wet, and he assured me he would dry me. He proceeded to do so, with a large bath towel, just as if I had been a child. Then he gave me a massage without a sheet in sight. He was completely professional and I was comfortable.

By contrast, when I had a massage back in the States, the masseuse showed me to a bed covered with sheets. She asked me to disrobe, get onto the bed, and then stepped out of the room while I did so. During the massage she exposed my back, my legs, and my arms, but never my whole body. When I asked her about it, and told her the story of the masseur in Germany, she looked surprised. I asked her if she was protecting my modesty, and she thought a while before saying, "I think I do it for myself."

Why is it all right if nudity and sex are fantasy, and not all right if they are real? Why is it acceptable for whole families to bathe together in Japan, for Spanish tourists to tan topless at the Costa del Sol, for German women to enjoy mineral springs without bathing suits, but not for American women to be seen nude? Why do we allow American children to be titillated by every variety of nudity in the media, and then tell them, "Not for you, kids. Just say 'No!'"? It's our attitude, our double standard concerning sexuality.

Because of their upbringing, European youngsters know it's not polite to stare at topless sunbathers and they don't. They also know that sex involves respect and responsibility. If they are sexually active, they use contraception accordingly.

When I recently taught a teen mother class in Florida, I proposed to the teachers that I show a European video of "Safe Sex or No Sex" commercials. When the teachers previewed the video, one expressed concern about what might happen if the parents heard about it. I held a discussion with the students, but did not show them the video.

"What do you mean?" one teen mom asked after I had de-scribed the video. "Do you mean they actually show people getting undressed and getting ready for sex?"

I responded, "Yes, they do that. Then they make a point of showing a condom, and of letting the viewer know that if there is no condom, there is no sex. One partner will stop it. That's because the message is respect and responsibility."

She was horrified, saying that sex was too private to be shown in public that way. She wouldn't have sex on the public street.

"Is TV like a public street?" I asked.

"Yes," she said.

The other teen was as heated in her discussion. "Are you crazy?" she asked. "Don't we see far worse things in movies, on the soaps, on MTV, and in ads? The only difference is we never see condoms or the message that tells about safe sex. So what are you against, the sex or the condoms?"

Comparing Teen Births, Abortion, HIV/AIDS

In the three European countries study tour participants visited, we observed and heard about far different attitudes toward nudity and sexuality. We also saw a much more positive acceptance of adolescents as young people to be respected and trusted. Adults don't appear to see adolescents as "problems" as often happens in the United States. Rather, we were told, "Our children and our young people are our greatest asset. We cherish and respect them."

Whatever the attitudinal differences in these European countries, the teen birth, abortion, and AIDS rates are extremely different when compared with the United States:

Birth, Abortion, HIV/AIDS Data
United States, France, Germany, Netherlands[3]

	Teen Births per 1,000 women ages 15-19	Teen Abortions per 1,000 women ages 15-19	HIV/AIDS per 1,000 for all ages	Average Age Initiation of Sexual Intercourse
France	9	8.9	4.8	16.6
Germany	14	3.1	1.7	17.4
Netherlands	4	4.2	2.2	17.7
United States	51	26.8	21.7	16.3

The Netherlands has the lowest rate in teen births and the highest age for initiation of sexual intercourse. Germany has the lowest rate of HIV/AIDS and the lowest teen abortion rate. The United States loses in all categories. Compared to the Netherlands, the U.S. has, per 1000 teens, thirteen times the rate of teen births and more than six times as many abortions. The HIV/AIDS rate per 1000 of all ages is nearly ten times higher in the United States than in the Netherlands.

The United States is the only country in this group to advocate sexual abstinence for youth. The statistics show, however, that U.S. teens initiate sexual intercourse *earlier* than in any of these other countries, actually almost one and one-half years earlier than they do in the Netherlands.

Allowing for Different Populations

Comparing a country as small and homogeneous as the Netherlands with the far larger and heterogeneous United States is difficult. Perhaps comparing birth and abortion data along with area and population of specific states can help. Note that some states here (as well as the District of Columbia), are smaller than the Netherlands.

Comparison of Birth and Abortion Data[4, 5]

	Area in Sq.Mi.	Population	Births per 1000 15-19	Abortions per 1000 15-19
The Netherlands	**16,033**	**15,653,091**	**4**	**4.2**
New Hampshire	8,969	1,185,048	29	20
Vermont	9,249	590,883	27	22
Massachusetts	7,939	6,147,132	32	37
New Jersey	7,419	7,730,118	35	50
New York	47,224	18,175,301	39	53
Tennessee	41,220	5,430,621	65	18
Georgia	57,919	7,642,207	67	25
Mississippi	46,914	2,752,092	74	16
Wisconsin	54,314	5,223,500	36	15
Missouri	68,898	5,438,559	52	19
Idaho	82,751	1,163,261	47	12
Arizona	113,642	4,668,631	70	27
California	155,973	32,666,550	57	45
District of Columbia	68	523,124	102	NA

At first glance these statistics show us that even our state with the lowest population, Vermont, with 1/26 as many people as the Netherlands, has seven times the teen birth rate. Our highest state, Mississippi, one-fifth the population of the Netherlands, has eighteen times the teen birth rate. And the District of Columbia, with a population less than 1/30 of the Netherlands, has a teen birth rate 25 times higher! The abortion rate among teens in each state is far higher, too.

Two other contributing factors need to be compared: the homogeneity of European versus American societies as well as the affluence/poverty factors.

Even with all their success, the Dutch are finding that as different cultures emigrate to the Netherlands, they face issues they never had before. Some of their new émigrés are fundamentalist in their views, and the Dutch sexuality educators are having a hard time reaching the young of new immigrants, especially the boys.

Ethnic Distribution[6]

(By percentage of females aged 15-19)

	White	African American	Hispanic	Asian Pacific Islands	Native Americans	Other
*The Netherlands	95					** 5
New Hampshire	96	<1	2	1		
Vermont	96	1	1	1	<1	
Massachusetts	80	7	8	4	1	
New York	60	17	18	5		
Tennessee	76	21	2	<1	<1	
Georgia	60	35	3	2	<1	
Michigan	52	46	<1	<1	<1	
Wisconsin	87	7	3	2	1	
Missouri	83	14	2	1	<1	
Idaho	87	<1	10	1	1	
Arizona	59	4	28	2	7	
California	42	8	38	11	1	
District of Columbia	13	75	8	3	<1	

* Percentage for total population. (State data refers to females aged 15-19 only.)

** First generation immigrants from Morocco, Turkey, Surinam, Dutch Antilles

New Hampshire is little more than half the size of the Netherlands. The population of the state is slightly over one million compared to more than fifteen million in the Netherlands. It has

an even higher proportion of white residents than the
Netherlands does. New Hampshire also has the lowest percentage of people living below the poverty line (7.7 percent) of any
state in the United States. Yet even New Hampshire has *seven*
times the number of teen births and almost *five* times the number
of abortions per 1000 as does the Netherlands. Excusing the high
rates of teen births and abortion in the United States on the basis
of size, ethnic make-up, and poverty alone is not a valid
argument.

Impact of Poverty on Teen Pregnancy

The Netherlands is considered an affluent country, while the
United States, in spite of a surging economy, has large pockets of
poverty, particularly among the urban and rural young.

In 1997, according to *Time Almanac 2000,* 10.9 percent of
United States residents were living in poverty. The poverty
threshold was based on an income of $16,400 for a family of
four. Almost twice that many children under 18, 19.9 percent,
were living below the poverty level. Although children represent
only 25 percent of the total population, they represent 40 percent
of the poor population.[7]

As the poverty rate rises, we generally see higher birth rates,
except in those states that also have high abortion rates. (See
chart on the opposite page.) The solution would seem to lie first
in the alleviation of poverty, then in the prevention of pregnancy,
resulting in the prevention of the need for abortion.

If we are tempted to point a finger at the African American
community, let's look at the statistics. In 1991 the teen (15-19)
birth rates per thousand were: Caucasian, 43; African American,
115; Hispanic, 107. By 1998, the birth rates had dropped:
Caucasian, 38; African American, 91; Hispanic, 102. This shows
a decline of 13 percent for Caucasians, 5 percent for Hispanics,
and 21 percent for African Americans.[8]

As the economy has improved over the last five years, and as
joblessness has decreased, we have seen a sharper decline in the
African American birth rate than in any other group. Some of the
contributing factors: less poverty, more access to injectable

Poverty Levels by State
Compared with Teen Birth and Abortion Rates[9, 10]
(From Lowest to Highest Poverty Level)

	Percent Below Poverty Line	Teen Births per 1000 15-19 years	Abortions per 1000 15-19 years	Births Plus Abortions
The Netherlands	**Affluent**	**4**	**4.2**	**8.2**
New Hampshire	7.7	29	20	49
Wisconsin	8.5	36	15	51
Missouri	10.6	52	19	71
Vermont	10.9	27	22	49
Massachusetts	11.2	32	37	69
Idaho	13.3	43	12	55
Georgia	14.7	67	25	92
Tennessee	15.1	65	18	83
New York	16.6	39	53	92
California	16.8	57	45	102
Mississippi	18.6	74	16	90
Arizona	18.8	70	27	97
District of Columbia	23.0	102	NA	NA

contraceptives and condoms, fear of AIDS, and a growing acceptability of the idea of contraception.

Teens — A Breed Apart

In addition to their problems caused by poverty and cultural heterogeneity, U.S. adolescents face discrimination just because of their age. This attitude is reflected in all ways, not only in conflicts about sexuality education. They are singled out as "teenagers," a breed apart, rather than as "our young people," as they are affectionately called in Europe.

Mike Males, author of *The Scapegoat Generation,* makes these points.[11] Although adults think teens are everywhere and into every kind of trouble, Males cites this data:

• Teens are poorer than they used to be.

• Grownups have more deaths from drugs, compared to teens.

• More adults are mentally disturbed.

• Only ten percent of crime is committed by adolescents.

• Of all single mothers giving birth, only 30 percent were under 20.[12]

Teen poverty is caused by adult-decreed financial means-tested programs to provide benefits. Wealthy elders seem unwilling or unable to raise benefits high enough to move people out of poverty. They provide no safety net. What seniors don't understand is that how well they live depends on how well younger people are doing. Even if elders don't wish to protect young people from poverty for altruistic reasons, they might consider doing it for their own self-interest.[13]

Adults claim that in the name of safety they must protect youth from alcohol, guns, employment, speech, sexual behaviors, driving, and access to media. Yet they permit themselves nearly absolute freedom in these areas. If all this is for "safety," why not for adults as well?[14] Votes about education, welfare, taxation, immigrants' rights, and civil rights nearly always split along youth/adult lines. Why are we at war with one another rather than seeing each other as members of the same family?

"We must reclaim them as our own," says Males.[15]

Lessons Learned in Europe

The European Study Tour of 1998, followed by similar tours in 1999 and 2000, offered participants opportunities to learn reasons behind statistics on teen births, abortion, HIV/AIDS, and age for initiation of sexual intercourse. According to Berne and Huberman, "The lessons learned on these tours can have valuable implications for U.S. efforts to improve the sexual health of adolescents." They describe these lessons as follows:[16]

• The Dutch, Germans, and French view young people as assets, not as problems. They value and respect adolescents and expect teens to act responsibly. Governments strongly support education and economic self-sufficiency for youth.

• The morality of sexual behavior is weighed through an

individual ethic that includes the values of responsibility, love, respect, tolerance, and equity. The morality of sexual behavior is not the result of collective force, such as religious dogma.

- Families, educators, and healthcare providers have open, honest, consistent discussions with teens about sexuality.

- Adults see intimate sexual relationships as normal and natural for older adolescents, a positive component of emotionally healthy maturation. Young people believe it is "stupid and irresponsible" to have sex without protection and use the maxim, "Safe sex or no sex."

- Marriage is not a criterion for intimate sexual relationships for older adolescents.

- The major impetus for improved access to contraception, consistent sexuality education, and widespread public education campaigns is a national desire to reduce the number of abortions and to prevent HIV infection.

- Sexually active youth have free, convenient access to contraception through national health insurance.

- Sexuality education is not necessarily a curriculum; it may be integrated through many school subjects and at all grade levels. Educators provide accurate and complete information in response to students' questions.

- Governments support massive, consistent, long-term public education campaigns utilizing television, films, radio, billboards, discos, pharmacies, and healthcare providers. Media is a partner, not a problem, in these campaigns. Sexually explicit campaigns arouse little concern.

- Research is the basis for public policies to reduce pregnancies, abortions, and STIs.

- Political and religious interest groups have little influence in public health policy.

Advice and Counsel from the Netherlands

Why was the Netherlands able to move from the Sexual
Revolution of the sixties to its progressive and effective policies
of the nineties, while we in the United States appear to have
moved in the opposite direction? Dr. Jany Rademakers, Research
Coordinator at NISSO (Netherlands Institute for Social Sexological Research), shares her views through her lens of distance
and experience.

I met with Dr. Rademakers in Washington, where we were
attending the follow-up to the study tour. I asked her to compare
our two countries and to talk about the conflicts we are facing
here. I wanted to know about the impact of religion on policies
in the Netherlands, and about the differences she sees in our
cultures. I asked her to make some recommendations for us.

"The Netherlands in the fifties and early sixties was similar in
a lot of respects to the American society right now, especially
regarding sexuality," Dr. Rademakers began. "That was the time
before we had the pill, before abortions were possible, a time
also in the Netherlands when we had the idea of people remain-
ing virgins until marriage. There were a lot of influences and
changes: the feminist group, women who wanted contraception,
women who wanted access to abortion, and the pill.

"There were also changes in the kind of political structure and
student influence in the universities, on programs, on classes, on
students having to be represented on all kinds of boards in
universities. It's a country where people may have influence
from the bottom up so it's a different idea about power. Very
important in the 70s and 80s was that religion became less
influential in society as a whole. Religion was more important
before that time. That started to change at the end of the sixties
just like it did in a lot of countries."

Dr. Rademakers compared the homogeneity of the Netherlands with our heterogeneity. "Five percent of our population are
first generation immigrants. This percentage goes to 16 percent if
you count everyone who has some heritage other than Dutch, so
we are not as homogeneous as we used to be," she pointed out.

"We're very busy trying to integrate the new people," she

continued. "It is difficult sometimes because the Islamic, especially the males, are so opposed to the Dutch ideas about sexuality and homosexuality. The immigrant boys are opposed to premarital sex and homosexuality. We want to respect their values, but when we teach sex education, we feel strongly that we must teach the values of respect and responsibility for everyone."

Dr. Rademakers acknowledged that because of this immigration with its different culture, they now have a religious right emerging. They are trying to understand it by researching the attitudes and beliefs of this different culture so that they will be able to deal with this change.

Her comments shed some light on our difficulties. However, our problems related to teen sexuality are much greater, partly due to the relative size of the two countries as well as to the number and variety of immigrants.

Could Dr. Rademakers help us find our way? She suggested, "Don't try to change the whole country over night. We've been working on it for forty years. In America everything is big and fast. I think the way to do this is from the inside out, trying to convince people, the little people, the school boards, the teachers, and the administrators who see the possibilities and who will make change. Start from the inside out and show others that change can happen.

"Be sure to evaluate what you do. It is important for people to see what has been done about adolescent sexual health. This is very important in your country, to show that it works. People who are very sensitive to money, show them the benefits, show that it saves money. This will work better instead of trying to do it from the top down.

"Look at your states that are exemplary, and focus on them as examples of where it is working. Look at your more open states and let them show the other states. Empower teachers who are willing, but afraid."

We Are All Afraid

Many of us are afraid. Three high school administrators in Florida refused to give out a survey I sent them. The survey asked teens anonymously about their sexual attitudes and behaviors. It also asked them if they thought a media campaign like that in the Netherlands would have changed their lives in any way. The administrators each said that they would like to distribute the survey but their school boards did not approve.

Teachers are afraid. I spoke at a teen pregnancy prevention conference in Tennessee last year and told them about the policies in the Netherlands. After I recommended that we initiate such policies in our country, teachers came up to talk with me privately. They worry that Tennessee has one of the highest rates of teen births in the country, and they thanked me for raising this issue publicly. Now they might finally begin to address it with their administrators and school boards.

Non-educators are afraid, too. The more liberal-thinking people are afraid that those who oppose teaching disease prevention and contraceptive methods along with abstinence will have the power to block their efforts. They're afraid that Congress will continue to fund Abstinence Only education (see chapter 7) and not continue programs like Title X, which gives access to reproductive health services to poor women and girls.

The more conservative people are afraid that their views will be ignored. They fear that comprehensive sexuality education will encourage premarital sex. They fear for the morality of the country as a whole, and of young people in particular.

I am reminded of the feeling I had when I was riding in a motor boat during a storm. On the wall of the cabin was a plaque that read, "Oh, Lord, thy sea is so great and my ship is so small!" That's how I feel now about the vastness of this country, about the wide abyss between opposing points of view regarding teen sexuality and pregnancy prevention, and about the enormity of the problems we have to address.

If we are to find workable solutions, we must make every effort *to understand all points of view, to overcome fear of the other, and to release our individual positions in order to embrace our mutual interests.*

CHAPTER

2

The Struggle
for Family Values

Sometimes values are in conflict. In Genesis, the Divine commission is to replenish the earth and that includes the parenting part of our human sexuality. You replenish the earth by having babies. We've done a pretty good job of it.

When is that commission fulfilled? We are struggling with that in the world community. Now the question is how are we responsible for our human sexuality in terms of childbirth? All of us are having to re-assess that in terms of birth control. Will there be a post-parent period when by necessity we will have to realize that human sexuality is not just for having children, but is for the creation of community between people?

Reverend Frank Hawkins, Tennessee

America cares about ethical choices. Americans care very much. The code words for caring have become, "We need to take back family values." But what are family values, who took them away, and what is it we want to take back? Most Americans do not have a strong leaning to either the left or the right. Many do not advocate either total freedom or total control. Regardless of political/religious leanings, most people agree that family values include respect, responsibility, interdependence, honesty, integrity, sharing, fairness, love, and nurturing, among others. It is helpful, however, to examine the points of view at either end of the values continuum in order to understand the extent of the conflict America faces today. Much of this diversity can be roughly divided into two categories:

One viewpoint, often considered socially conservative and/or religious fundamentalist, goes something like this. Before the Sexual Revolution of the sixties, and before the idea of freedom turned young people away from tradition, we had real family values. We need to take them back. Real family values are based on the literal teachings of Scripture:

• People are religious and church-going.

• Heterosexual couples marry and have children without birth control and with no thought of abortion.

• Young people abstain from sexual intercourse until marriage.

• Women submit to the authority of the man of the house.

• Both men and women submit to the authority of the Church.

In this view, these values are the true and only path. Being obedient and chaste are values. Abstaining from sex until marriage is a value. If we do all these things, we will have regained our family values and the problems of society will be cured.

Other people, sometimes labeled progressive, are dedicated to freedom of choice. Choosing well and wisely is a value. Their viewpoint goes something like this: During the Sexual Revolution of the sixties, the birth control pill gave people the opportunity to make more choices about their sexuality.

Democracy calls for us to be open to and accepting of alternative lifestyles and sexual orientation. Real family values are based on the principle that people have freedom of choice and the right to:

- Be religious or not.
- Choose abortion as an option.
- Receive comprehensive sexuality education including an understanding of both conception and contraception, as well as protection from disease.
- An education which inculcates responsibility and will make students knowledgeable enough to make wise choices.
- Access to family planning clinics for the prevention of pregnancy and sexually transmitted infections.
- A government-funded safety net for those who are unable to provide their own.
- Question authority, even that of religious tenets and of governmental control.

These are the family values that will address the ills of society, according to the more liberal viewpoint.

Conservatives and liberals agree we need to do something about teen pregnancy. Those in the first group see premarital sex as a moral issue, and are clear in their objection to it. "Be abstinent," they say. "This is the only sure way to protect yourself not only from pregnancy but from disease. This is the moral way to behave."

Others agree that delaying sex is advisable for adolescents. They base their thinking on the physical, emotional, and economic consequences of early sex rather than on the issue of morality. Many who consider themselves liberal agree that abstinence is the best form of contraception. If young people do not abstain, however, they are likely to say, "Be careful and respectful, not only about your body, but about your partner's. This is the responsible way to behave."

Defining Family Values

This disagreement, highly emotional and often political in nature, came to be known in the nineties as the issue of "family values." Americans are having as hard a time agreeing about what that means as they are about which values should prevail in our society.

What used to be a definition of family isn't so clear any more. The traditional model — a father, a mother, and some children — isn't the norm for all people, in fact, not for most families today. A family can consist of two partners, either heterosexual or homosexual, with or without children. Or a family can consist of a single parent and child(ren). Another family can be a group of non-related individuals who choose to live together and care for each other. A family can be three-generational, and it can be all women or all men. Families today come in all of these configurations, and in others as well.

We might more readily agree on the meaning of *values* as being something people use as guides for living. The problem then becomes which values we will follow. We are in conflict with each other, and sometimes within ourselves.

One of the common values in our society is love of money and what it can buy — success, fame, influence. No, say others, it's the hard work and what it can accomplish that we value. We say we value "character," especially honesty and integrity and the trust, friendship and influence such traits inspire. But don't we sometimes smile over someone's ability to outsmart the system, even if it takes a few short cuts to do it? Don't we appear to value that, too?

We value education, learning, and knowledge. Some care about these for their intrinsic value, and others for the good life they can foster. We value modesty but, at the same time, we value aggressiveness that is daring. We value the Bill of Rights and the Ten Commandments, though we may sometimes feel free to select only those precepts that fit best with our behaviors. We value independence and freedom, but we also value the characteristics of compliance and followership when useful for our purposes. Conflicts between us engender discussion, even argument, and we deal with those.

But what do we do when there is conflict within us? What do we do when our value of loyalty to our religious teachings conflicts with our value of loyalty to the well-being of ourselves and our children?

Why are our conflicts so intense, causing both private citizens and public legislators to lose their tempers with each other? Perhaps it has to do with how we develop values and the heavy, emotional component that goes with them. Values are taught by example; they are emulated. They are even developed by seeing things we don't like and vowing to be different.

Values Stir Emotions

Perhaps values stir emotions because "family" often conjures up hearth and home, a time when we were small and safe. "Values" presses buttons in our head, buttons that were implanted when we were part of that small, intimate group we lived with. We choose friends with similar values, and if we are lucky, we find mates who share our values.

"Thou shalt not steal." My mother was frowning, holding me by the hand, and leading me back to the Five and Ten Cent Store from which I had taken a hair clip I liked. She took me to the manager, told me to give it to him and apologize for taking it without paying for it. I was five and I still remember. A value.

"Always give something to charity for people who are not as fortunate as you," she said. We were standing beside the Blue Box that sat on a counter in our kitchen, a box that was for charity to Palestine, but I never knew what kind of charity. Even today, any box of any color, sitting on any counter, beckons me to open my purse and put some money in. A value.

"One hand washes another," she consoled me, after I had a fight with a friend. "You can catch more flies with honey." She talked about negotiating and being reasonable rather than getting angry. It feels better and it works better. Concern for others and pragmatism were born simultaneously. Values which conflict at times.

"First you work and then you play," said my father when I wanted to go out and play with my friends before I did my homework. Retired now, and punching the clock for no one, I seldom pick up a book to read or turn on the television until my work for that day is done. A value.

Sometimes, in our zeal to do the right thing, we are confused. "You *lied* to me," I said to our ten-year-old son. "You said you

didn't do . . . and you did." I was shattered, at the age of 39, to
think this perfect child would lie. In retrospect I see that if he'd
been completely comfortable with our unconditional acceptance
of him, even if his behavior was against the rules, he'd have told
the truth.

The value we had instilled was "Nice boys don't . . ." rather
than "You're always safe with us." Our family learned a new
value from that. True communication depends on trust. That
incident taught us to value trust above all.

Values and Ethics

Which are the "right" values?

If they are the ideals, the principles, the beliefs that our family
or our group cherishes and lives by — does that make them the
right ones? Are we talking about morality, about being good
people? about worshiping God or another higher being? about
caring for our fellow human beings? about diligence? about
cleanliness in mind and body? about loving? saving money?
being unselfish? doing unto others as you would have them do
unto you? obeying the rules of your religion? your family? your
government? Any or all of these could be your values, or they
could be someone else's. As we reflect critically on the problems
we face in the sexual arena today, and as we see valid ethical
considerations on both sides, perhaps ethical theory can help us
in our deliberations.

Ethicist Eugene Beam, Professor Emeritus at Baldwin
Wallace College in Ohio, explains it this way: "Ethics are a
matter of principle or a matter of consequences to society. When
you look at the numbers (comparing the United States teen birth
rate with the Netherlands), what can you say? As I see it, the
European attitude you describe meets the test of respect for
youth and the test of what's best for society. Ethical norms *are*
social norms."

Another philosopher, Emmanuel Kant, taught that rules for
virtuous human conduct do not necessarily depend on a
theological view of the world.[1] In other words, people can be
good and virtuous without being religiously oriented.

What does it mean to be "religious"? Sometimes the word is used in areas that have nothing to do with church attendance or religious ritual. Generally, though, the word has to do with believing in something and seriously attending to it. For example, people who exercise every day, never miss a session if at all possible, say they are "religious" in following their schedule. This is ritualized behavior as are lighting the Friday night candles, making the sign of the cross with holy water, or facing Mecca to pray.

So "religion," which surely means faith in a higher being, may also mean faith in other beliefs such as good health, love of fellow man, "Do unto others . . . ," and the medical mantra, "First of all, do no harm."

Kant's philosophy of Universality,[2] that one performs one's duty for the sake of duty and not for any other reason, is more in keeping with the moral stance of conservatives than it is with the stance of liberals. Yet both might agree that there are universals that guide everyone, i.e., the importance of treating people with the respect and moral dignity to which every person is entitled at all times. This could serve as the basis of a social policy that offers everyone equal access to and opportunity for reproductive healthcare. Whatever your first principles are, if they are aimed toward a "good," according to Kant, they may be virtuous conduct.

Beam points out that John Stuart Mill's famous Utilitarianism made an enormous impact on ethical thinking. Mill's premise was, "An act's rightness or wrongness resides in the results which the act brings about. Those acts are wrong (that) bring about bad or undesirable consequences." We talk about his idea today as "the greatest good for the greatest number."[3]

This theory was criticized by some as a "Godless doctrine" but defended by others who point out that "If God desires the happiness of His creatures, and if that was His purpose in their creation, Utility is . . . profoundly religious."[4] Since unwanted children, disease, and unnecessary abortion are not conducive to either individual or community happiness, can we not call avoidance of them a religious act?

Mind versus Heart

There is a big difference between philosophy and values. Theories are ideas that we can take or leave. They appeal to the mind. But values are embedded in the heart. Taking or leaving them is much harder. That's what make values so hard to change.

Lars Jonassen, a 46-year-old teacher and coach in Maine, calls for responsibility on the part of both the teens and the adults:

I like that part of it. I like the idea that the Dutch are saying, "It's up to you," and putting the responsibility on the kids. In our society neither kids nor adults take enough responsibility for what they do. That's what we need to teach.

Look at the statistics! Four per thousand compared with 51 here. It's unbelievable! They said their young people were their only resource. They put their money and effort into their development, and look how it's paid off. We blame the kids, but we're the ones who have to change.

Maybe "family values" is a misnomer. Perhaps it's parent values, or father values, or mother values, or church values, or government values, or, perhaps most important, one's own values. The one who decides the values is probably the one after whom they should be named. Does this imply that someone knows best? The more conservative view implies that someone certainly does; the more liberal view implies that each person needs to be properly educated in order to make wise personal decisions.

In the Netherlands, France, and Germany, children are taught by the media, by the schools, and by the society as a whole that if they are going to have a sexual relationship with another, they must consider the health and safety of each partner. They must not have children unless they are ready for a long term commitment that assures the care and safety of the child. They must not have sexual relations unless they take care to protect themselves and the other. And they must not rely on abortion or the morning after pill as birth control. They must use efficient contraceptive methods, preferably a condom in combination with the pill, the implant, or other female method. Thus, they are protected both from pregnancy and from STIs.

When this lesson is taught from the earliest ages on, the statistics for the age of initiation of sex, for unwanted children, for STIs and abortion show such positive results that American statistics in these areas appear tragic by comparison.

Yes, we must teach and model morality, a new morality that considers the health and safety of human beings. Not withholding, but reaching out. Not guilty of indiscretions, but proud of concern. Not berating unfaithfulness, but encouraging faithfulness to the ideal of caring for self, for each other, and for society as a whole.

Negotiating Areas of Disagreement

Values differ from one group to another, within families, and from one individual to another. Can we negotiate our values for the good of all? Which values are non-negotiable?

Any kind of anti-person behavior should be non-negotiable. In our great democracy, racism, homophobia, anti-Semitism, and acts against people because of their status or lack of it, should all be non-negotiable. We can't come to terms with them.

Invasion of privacy should be non-negotiable. The government should not delve into the issues of whether a woman or man of any age uses protection/contraception or with whom s/he chooses to live. The government should not control access to abortion. Public policy has no business in private matters between an individual and his/her partner, physician, or parents.

Out-of-control rage should be non-negotiable. It is not the best frame of mind in which to make any great decisions.

Moderates in the middle recognize these values and support them. They know that extreme positions do not work for society. Families without guidelines break up. Families with only guidelines become dysfunctional as well. So it is with societies.

The extremists do not support this reasoning. They believe the United States needs to swing to their end of the pendulum in order to regain moral authority. They are in direct opposition to each other.

The extremists on the right believe they will weed out the evil, the lying, the cover-ups, the misbehavior, the vulgarities, the political maneuvering, the dissembling. They will make America pure, virginal, clean, neat, honest, civil, well-behaved, scrubbed, and moral. Only through their route will we all come to be "good" again.

The extremists on the left support any law that means "freedom," no matter how irresponsible that may be. They will choose rights over responsibility, freedom of the individual over respect for the rules of society.

Hope for the future lies not in taking entrenched positions, but in seeking balance through negotiation. You don't have to be a "liberal" to be a centrist. The surest route to a functional, healthy, happy home, school, organization or group of organizations is through clear, fair, people-friendly policies backed by the vast numbers of people who occupy the moderate middle ground.

Can we change the definition of morality? Is it immoral to have unprotected sex? Is it immoral to have unwanted babies? Is it immoral to spread disease? Is it immoral to have an abortion when you could have prevented the conception in the first place? And is society immoral if it does not provide access to contraception in user-friendly clinics, if it does not provide early sex education, and if it does not remove stigma and judgment from teen sexuality?

Most Americans today understand both culturally and politically that it is time to take a fresh look at our social problems. They understand that access to contraception and the fight over the right to abortion are tied together. They know that we need to broaden the scope of our concern, gather around our mutual aversion to unwanted children, infections, and abortion, and eliminate the need by eliminating the causes. They realize *we must attack the problems, not the people.*

CHAPTER

3

Teen Sex —
What's a Parent to Do?

We had no sex education in church, and even though we had plenty in school, they didn't emphasize the results. We never went into sexually transmitted diseases and not much about contraception either. There was nothing about feelings, drives, hormones. It was strictly biological. But my mom talked with me about all these things all through my teen years, and that was real protection for me.

Now I can't always figure out what's going on with me biologically, but emotionally I can. I can relate to my emotions. When Mom spoke to me on that level about the feelings I would encounter, not just love, but lust and passion too, I understood because it was my feelings. So that's what really works.

Yolanda, 17, New York

Before we can address the real issues of teen pregnancy and sexually transmitted infections, we must take a look at the myth that permeates our perceptions of young people: parents don't matter, only their peers matter to teens.

Importance of Parental Guidance

The myth that parents don't matter to teens may be the most insidious of all. Parents who believe they make no difference in their adolescents' lives may choose to withdraw, give up, or otherwise disappear from the lives of their children just when they need them the most. Part of the coming of age syndrome is that teens must give the impression that they don't need their parents or respect their opinions. The truth is, the harder they fight to show their independence in order to become adults, the more they need to know their parents are there to guide and protect them when they need it.

The overwhelming majority of studies indicate that parent/child closeness is associated with reduced pregnancy risk. Teens who are close to their parents are more likely to remain sexually abstinent, postpone intercourse, have fewer sexual partners, and use contraception consistently.[1]

Do parents matter? Without a doubt. A sense of self, which comes from positive qualities exhibited by parents, is what takes a child into secure adolescence and adulthood.

Teens pay a lot of attention to peers as well, but caring, adult mentors plus quality education are two of the most important keys to making a difference in the prevention of teen pregnancy. Certainly parents are the original adult mentors — the crucial ingredient is the quality and quantity of the caring.

In a societal change modeled on the Dutch culture, society and parents become the mentors, creating the village approach to helping teens. The teens absorb the values of respect and responsibility through the massive educational campaigns of the media and the schools.

Then peers are saying the same things to each other that the messages are saying to all of them. The question of who matters more is a moot one. Both parents and peers matter. When the message they deliver is the same, teens are not confused and ambivalent.

Evolving Approach

In the Netherlands, France and Germany, most adults don't see teenage sex as a problem *if* protection is used. Parents accept youth as sexual beings. They realize that sexual intercourse is a logical part of intimate relationships. They support both abstinent and sexually active teens in making responsible decisions. The goal is for people to develop a *healthy* sexuality.

"It took fifteen to twenty years to get to today's level," says Dr. Jany Rademakers, Research Coordinator at NISSO (Netherlands Institute for Social Sexological Research). "In the early years most parents weren't comfortable with young people having sex, but they decided they would be doing it anyway, and what did parents want? The people of the Netherlands accepted that many adolescents will have sexual intercourse whether they liked it or not."

This is not Europe. In America you don't have to be a social or religious conservative to be uncomfortable with the idea of adolescents having sex. It's a different concept for most Americans. The European countries we visited left their discomfort behind when they made their vast social changes in the sixties. Their motivation to lower abortion rates, unplanned pregnancies and sexually transmitted infections was strong enough to overcome their judgmentalism about youthful sex.

"Abstinence is not a topic on its own," Dr. Rademakers continued. "We talk with young people about waiting until you're sure it's what you want, what your partner wants, and if you're ready. We did have Abstinence Until Marriage in the fifties, with shotgun weddings, but not anymore. In the Netherlands we don't have good girls who don't have sex and bad girls who do. We have bad girls who don't use contraception.

"In the Netherlands we had change from the bottom up. The parents' wishes worked to influence government policy. Government didn't take the lead, but it reflected and followed the people. Certain people in the field were busy spreading their ideas and, like drops of oil, they spread and got bigger. Then it became policy.

"In the United States there is a discrepancy between what

people want and what the government does. Policy comes from
the top down. There is a collective Puritanism about intercourse.
Some people are afraid of it. Others have to convince them. They
have to convince each other, then the school boards, then local
politicians. It has to go from the bottom up."

Dutch, German, and French parents use multiple channels to
ensure that teens are well informed and socially skilled, and they
may provide teens with condoms and contraception to protect
themselves. Parents then trust teens to make good choices for
themselves and to be responsible, according to Dr. Rademakers.

In the United States there isn't the same consensus about
what's good for young people. Many young people and their
parents do not have honest, open communication regarding
sexuality. Many young people don't receive much parental or
community support or information about respect, intimate
relationships, responsible decision making, and about the absolute need for protection in sexual relationships. Teens who feel
connected to a parent are protected against health risks including
early sexual activity.[2]

A really difficult area for many Americans is premarital sex
for adolescents. According to *Sex and America's Teenagers*,
"One third of teens surveyed said they thought (premarital sex)
was a mistake because of the danger of AIDS and the possibility
of pregnancy, while two-thirds said it was all right to have sex
before marriage. None expressed a moral aversion."[3] The teens
were echoing the adult attitudes and statistics when asked this
question.

Parents as *First* Teachers

From the beginning children learn from their parents. Parents,
as their children's first educators, are surely the most important.
Some are both knowledgeable and comfortable enough to talk
with their children about sexuality and guide them through their
adolescent years. Most are not. Some parents deny both their
own sexuality and that of their children.

Just as children whose parents are comfortable with their
sexuality learn to be comfortable, so do children of parents who

are uncomfortable learn to be uncomfortable. Sex can be a good thing or a bad thing.

Back of the home in which we raised our children was a wonderful 20' x 20' brick building we called the Summer House. Depending on our stage of life, we used it for everything from a playhouse for children to a party room for adults, to a storeroom for our summer camp. One day when our preschool children had been playing in the Summer House with their friends, I got a call from the mother of two of the boys. "The children were playing doctor at your Summer House. They may never play with your children again!" She told her little boys, aged five and six, that our children were now off limits. I doubt she told them why, but they had to surmise they had been doing something wrong.

Playing doctor, our children told us when we asked them, involved listening to heartbeats, using Popsicle sticks for oral thermometers, and examining each other's bodies to see the differences. We assured them that this curiosity was a normal part of growing up. The lesson their friends learned was that bodies are bad, examining them is worse, and being curious about ourselves is forbidden. That's sex ed that would be hard to forget.

According to Dr. James J. Jaccard of the University at Albany, State University of New York, parents' perceptions are not always the reality. Both those with the best relationships with their children and those who are the most critical are likely to underestimate the sexuality activity of their children. Almost all parents think they talk with their children about birth control, but only half of their teens say that they do.

Why the discrepancy? As every parent knows, just because we talk doesn't mean they hear. Another reason teens said they hadn't discussed sex with their parents might be that although parents think they are communicating about topics like birth control in relationships, they may be skirting the issue. Parents may use language that flirts with, but doesn't really address, the topic. They may be talking either above their children's heads or below their level of understanding. None of this constitutes good communication with anyone, let alone with teens, who may not want to hear it in the first place.

"You can talk to me," parents may tell their preteens and teens. "Feel free to come to me if you decide to have sex. I will help you and will get you protection." And then they feel very good because they think they have protected their children.

Listen to the story Stephanie told a group of public health workers I was interviewing. Stephanie, 46, has a daughter who is now 30. When Stephanie was fifteen her mother said, "You can come to me and tell me if you're going to have sex." Nevertheless, she felt her mother's disapproval. And besides, the 21-year-old she was dating told her not to worry. He would use the withdrawal method. So she had sex without telling her mother. With no knowledge about contraception either from her home or from the school, she became pregnant.

"If Mom had also told me about contraception and how to get it without her, I think that would have worked for me," she said.

The other public health workers agreed. "Yes, you can talk to your kids and you should, but this doesn't mean they will talk to you," they said. It isn't enough to be available for them. You must also be sure they have information about and personal access to contraception without your involvement. We can't assume that just because we say we're ready to listen, they're ready to talk.

Erin, 30, talked about her mother, a public health nurse, who understood this. "She knew who was pregnant even when we didn't, and she knew how kids thought," said this young woman.

"I have condoms in my office," the mother told her daughter, her son, and her son's girlfriend. "Go there when I'm not there and help yourself." Evidently it worked, for this young woman was not a teen mother.

Some parents don't talk to their children about sex at all. Dr. Jaccard suggests several reasons:

- They don't think they will have impact.
- They think they can't influence either the genes or the hormones.
- They think their children will say they already know all that.
- They think it may be embarrassing to the adolescent and/or

themselves.
• They may be asked something they can't or don't want to
answer.

Dr. Jaccard makes a case for educating parents so that they
can do a good job of educating their children. He lists the
important variables in contraceptive use behavior — knowing
the choices, understanding the methods, choosing one or two
consciously, and using them with consistency.

In spite of recent books to the contrary, parents have a great
deal of influence, he says, and there is a growing body of research that shows that parents not only make a difference, but
can have a very significant impact on adolescents. Parents have
the advantage, unlike teachers, of being with their children
through each stage of development. Teaching them about
contraception can be part of the values they teach.

An interesting statistic from the United States: Teens who
think they know it all are the ones most likely to end up
being pregnant.

Common Sense Tips for Parents

Parents who want to protect their children may not be sure
they know how. The National Campaign to Prevent Teen
Pregnancy offers parents ten tips to help them.[4]

The first tip, and the most important, is to be clear about your
values first. The booklet asks, "What do you really think about
school-aged teenagers becoming sexually active?" "What do you
think about teenagers using contraception?" It's easier to talk
with your children about sex, love, and relationhips if you know
what your values are.

Talk early and often. Make sure your conversations are
between you, not you talking at your children. Be honest and
respectful. A scene you have both seen in a movie or on TV can
be a good conversation starter.

These suggestions are built on a close, strong relationship
with your children. Mutual trust and respect are at the core.
Supervise them, know their friends and discourage early dating.

Take a strong stand against a daughter dating a boy significantly older. In fact, *all* adolescents should be encouraged to date someone close in age. Make their future look bright by talking about goals and valuing education. Control the media in your home and let them know your views about media depictions of casual sex without consequences.

Most of all, express your love. Show your children courtesy and respect and expect them in return. It's all common sense, but it's comforting to know that research says it works.

Parents Are Conflicted

The conflict *between* groups advocating for comprehensive sexuality education (Abstinence Plus) and those advocating for Abstinence Only education are a reflection of the types of conflict *within* some people.

Jim and Julie, a couple in their forties, live in a small community outside Boston. Both parents work at home, and their children are 15, 13, and 6. Their responses to the following questions reveal the conflict they're feeling regarding their children's sexuality:

"What do you want your teenagers to know about sexuality?"

Julie: *I feel they should know a lot and I want them to have a positive attitude. I don't want them to feel pushed into sex when they aren't ready for it. I like to keep the lines of communication open. Sex is a great thing when you're ready, not when you're not.*

"What should schools be teaching in sexuality education classes?"

Julie: *We have a great program here that begins in fifth grade. Some parents thought it was too early, but I think it's perfect. They are old enough to retain the information, and it catches them before they begin to develop. Schools can get into feelings during freshman year in high school.*

"At what age do you think it's appropriate for teens to have sex?"

Julie: *I'm kind of conservative about that. I told my daughter I'd like her to wait until college. Her mind and body will develop more after high school.*

"Do you think parents can make a difference?"

Julie: *Definitely. They need to let children know they remember their feelings when they were growing up. They need to form parents' networks. Parents need to let each other know how they feel about curfews, things like that. Parents need to be with their kids, drive them around, listen to what they talk about, get to know their friends, bring up subjects with them. They need to give their opinions on things.*

Jim: *Parents get report cards. They work with their children from birth until puberty and beyond, and then the day comes when the young person goes out and does things on her/his own. They come back with body piercing, but they come back okay. The parent gets a B+. But you're still doing fine. The fear factor isn't a bad thing either. I mean letting your children know that their reputations depend on their behavior. The labels are out there in high school. If you're loose, especially girls, it gets out and you're labeled. It can't hurt for them to worry about that.*

"What about the media? What role should they have?"

Julie: *They could have public service announcements about sexually transmitted infections, but it's hard to put condoms on a billboard! I get conflicted because on the one hand you want to be open, understanding and approachable. On the other hand, you don't want to push them into sex before they're ready. Well, maybe the billboards would be all right. I guess it's okay.*

Jim and Julie are good parents. They are open and honest with their children. They let their children know they love them. They make time for them and they want them to have as much information as they need. They have some reservations about their teens being pushed into sex too early. They encourage them to wait until they graduate high school before they have intercourse. They want them to be "ready."

If you are a parent of teens or have any kind of a mentoring relationship with young people, ask yourself the questions I asked Jim and Julie:

1. What do you want your teenagers to know about sexuality?
2. What should the schools teach?
3. What should the family teach?
4. What should the role of the following institutions be?
   a. the church (temple, mosque, etc.)
   b. the government
   c. healthcare personnel
   d. the media
5. How influential do you think peers are?
6. At what age do you think it's appropriate for teens to have sexual intercourse?
7. Do you think parents (mentors) can make a difference?

Parents themselves may not know how powerful their influence is. When I asked a mother and daughter the questions above, their answers were revealing. The mother said, "Peers are the most influential. We pop in as visitors once in a while, but it's their world."

The daughter wondered aloud, and ended her deliberations with, "I think my mother has more influence."

Where do you fit? It's easy to break the sexuality education debate into two camps, the conservative and the liberal. But people don't fall so easily into one category. Jim and Julie are socially liberal, but they have United States conservative views about their own children's sexual involvement. They also recognize that we don't have a community/country consensus. About using billboards to advertise safer sex, Julie says, "At least they would have a consistent message." Jim points out to his daughter that she has a reputation to worry about.

What do you think?

CHAPTER
4

Influenced
by the Media

Look at what we do today. From 12 noon to 3 in the afternoon we have soap operas that push all kinds of pre-marital sex. If we're going to let that stuff be on TV, shouldn't we also have commercials that push contraception and responsibility?

I know nature is at work with young people, but they should be taught about the responsibility you take on when you conceive a child. If you want to spare kids grief, you should have the guts to say this is how to prevent an unwanted pregnancy.

Chuck Giallombardo, 53, barber-stylist, Florida

The Netherlands, France and Germany utilize the power of the media to ensure sexual responsibility. Our media could play this powerful role. In the European nations studied, a major public health goal is to ensure that everyone, including adolescents, has the necessary skills to behave responsibly when sexually active. Mass media campaigns are developed and delivered to educate entire populations. These campaigns encourage open and frank discussions about sexuality. Such discussions, they believe, contribute to the acceptance of sexuality as a normal and healthy component of life.[1]

Our media messages do not instill responsibility. TV sit-coms, for example, epitomize the free-sex-with-no-responsibility mindset. Those of us who used to worry so much about peer pressure on our children now realize that media pressure is by far the more important influence on their hearts and minds. People throng to toy stores for the latest fad advertised on TV. Telephone hot-lines lie cold when teens are glued to the final episode of a popular soap. It's hard to think of life without television in our homes.

What a love/hate affair Americans have with the media! Many of us can't live with them and we can't live without them. The media appear to be the single most influential part of our culture. People have grumbled about this influence since the advent of the printing press. My first recollection of adult concern about children and media was in 1935 when my dad, observing his three daughters lying on the floor glued to "The Phantom" on the radio, told my mother that the radio would ruin the children. How innocent it was then, but he could see the hold this fantasy show had on us.

My in-laws, well into middle age and after many years of marriage, came close to breaking up on an early September day in 1948 when the men, led by my father-in-law, refused to come to Rosh Hashanah dinner. The World Series between the Cleveland Indians and the Boston Braves was on TV in the other room. Move the TV to the dining room? Not on your life, stamped mother. Resolution? We brought the meal to the men in the game room and the women had dinner together in the dining room. I should have known then and there that we were in for a cultural revolution of the electronic kind.

Some of us remember the first sets mounted in store windows where people gathered on the street watching a black and white monitor together. Bars were frequented by sports enthusiasts having a beer and cheering on their favorite football team. Even then Americans were falling in love with TV.

No Escape from Media Messages

Picture two teens today, one living in a small rural town and the other in a large industrial city. No matter where or how teens live, they are exposed to our media culture. If they had been teens in the fifties, each would have been exposed to different kinds of experiences, but they are teens in the twenty-first century. Even if their financial and personal circumstances are very different, it is almost certain they have been exposed to the same media messages. Almost all have television sets. Many use the internet. They go to the movies. They listen to music. They see the covers of magazines, and they read the insides.

This culture is filled with sexual innuendo, steamy sex scenes. No messages tell teens that casual sex is not good for them. On the contrary, the scenes they see either on TV, in the print media, or in the movies sell sex to them. So do the lyrics of the music they hear. There is almost never a word about responsibility and the dangers of HIV, AIDS, and other sexually transmitted infections, or the problems they will face if they have an unplanned, unintended pregnancy.

In my supermarket, I saw these articles promoted on the covers of magazines at the checkout counter: "Supersize Your Sex Life: Massage Him, Knead Him, Totally Please Him — Three Magical Things Your Fingers Can Do" and "Sex He'll Never Forget — His Thighs Will Sizzle." These were not *Playboy* or *Hustler* — these were in "women's magazines."

The media folks are not only fighting for the hearts of teens; they are fighting for their wallets. They want teen dollars, and, knowing all about teens' wishes and fears, they sell wanting and having. They sell immediate gratification. They sell fun and popularity. They do it through depictions of passionate sex and through fear of rejection. If the teen doesn't respond to the "in" messages about dress and behavior, he or she may feel left out, a leftover, a loser. But if they do respond, happiness is in their hands. They can have it all. The message? *Just Do It!*

Television Affects Us All

Adults are agitated about these media messages. Tipper Gore, the wife of the U.S. vice president (2000), writes a book about the violent lyrics in some popular music and their influence on children. People join together to require TV to code its shows. Organizations give awards to programs and programmers who try to send positive and healthy messages to teens. In informal settings, people at parties, at parent-teacher meetings, and in doctors' offices complain about the effect of the media on the impressionable young.

It's time for us to control our emotions about TV and use our minds instead. The media, and TV in particular, are influencing teen sexuality in all the wrong ways. I feel a little like I did as a parent of teens when we didn't like the influence our children's friends were having on our children. We did everything parents do from telling them to see them less, to not seeing them at all, but we knew it was a losing battle.

It's the same with TV. We can rant and rave all we like, but children are watching it between three and five hours a day. That's close to the amount of time they spend in school, and surely more than they spend talking with their parents, or reading books, or playing sports, or doing things together as a family. We're talking about real influence, and it's up to us to make sure it's good for our children, not bad for them.

So much of it is bad for them. The Kaiser Family Foundation studied 1,351 TV programs between October, 1997, and March, 1998.[2] They found that 56 percent of the shows contained sexual content and averaged more than three scenes with sex per hour. Fifty percent of the scenes showed passionate kissing, twelve percent were scenes in which intercourse was strongly implied, and three percent depicted intercourse.

Even more important for impressionable teens is the fact that only nine percent of these shows discussed or showed contraception or mentioned risk.

The federal government is also aware that young people spend a lot of time in front of TV. To combat some of the pressure from parent groups, it has encouraged the networks to devote at least three hours a week to educational programming.[3] Networks appear willing to comply, but they know more about teen viewing habits than the government does. They are fearful that, with "educational" programming, they will be building "big black holes" in schedules because teens like irreverent humor, violence, and entertainment.

Teens don't like education on TV unless it is packaged as entertainment. Even then, it had better be sophisticated and savvy or they will change channels or turn it off as fast as they turn it on.

Programmers know that they need to package educational programs the same way they package the soaps, the teen programs, and the ads that young people love. This doesn't always happen.

Fantasy Promoted by Media and Government

Teens, who are in the stage of life where they have trouble just deciding who they are, are getting mixed messages about sex from two powerful influences, the media and the government. The media messages repeat:

"Just do it!"

"Buy this perfume and you'll be irresistible!"

"Wear these jeans and no man can keep his hands off you!"

"Drive this car and no woman can resist you."

"Wear this deodorant and you'll entice every male in sight!"

According to both research and our own observations, almost none of the ads or programs that either imply sex or show sex indicate the use of a condom.

At the same time, federal grants in the millions are given to states to convince teens to abstain, without providing education about contraceptive practices in case they don't abstain. (See chapter 7.) In those classes the emphasis is on condom or contraceptive failures, not successes, and students get no encouragement to use them.

Then television and other media, which make sex look like a really great idea, ignore protection entirely, so once again condoms are given no credibility. Two influential parts of children's lives — Abstinence Only sexuality education classes and media programs — and neither touches safer sex, disease prevention, or pregnancy prevention. First, teens hear that abstinence is the only acceptable way when they know it's not the reality for over half of them or even their parents. At the same time, they figure that unprotected sex has no consequences. Not much respect or responsibility here.

We know the media have a job to do. So does the American public. Viewers need to become media-literate. Parents and schools need to sensitize children to the covert advertising and programming messages they are receiving. When they see a perfume ad on TV, they may not recognize that what the ad is really selling is sex. Use this perfume and you will attract men. When they see an ad for a new car, they may not realize that the ad is really selling freedom from responsibility. In this car you will fly away from the real world. You can drive fast and there are no consequences.

The overt message may be the perfume or the car, but the covert message is what reaches the viewer. Once young people understand how ads work, they will be much wiser consumers. While we are waiting for the media to change, we can undo some of the damage by educating the viewers to the tactics advertisers use.

Most parents are squeamish about getting into sexual ethics, so teens seem to be making up the rules for themselves. They are patching together ideas from television shows, movies, music, magazines, and talk with their friends. Most get information from each other rather than from adults, and most don't have clear, real information to transmit. It's a vicious cycle — one that we have to stop by providing the kind of information and guidance teens need, and say they want.

As consumers of media products, we have a responsibility. First we have to tell the media that we recognize their power to influence young people. Second, we have to let them know that we object to their sensational, irresponsible depictions of sex. Finally, we have to convince them to use that power to deliver clear, consistent messages about sexual health.

TV Can Be Positive

Research results also support the positive influence of television. The Kaiser Foundation surveyed regular "ER" viewers between March 31, 1997 and June 30, 1997.

Learning that the April 10 episode would include mention of emergency contraception, they did their survey of 400 viewers at that time. In the show there is a vignette about a patient who has been the victim of a date rape, and who requests information about what she can do to prevent pregnancy. The mention of using birth control pills for post-coital contraception is less than a minute long in the segment. The researchers decided to see if there was a difference in awareness of emergency contraception before the viewing, directly after the viewing, and two months later. The results:[4]

- "The number of viewers who knew that a woman has options for prevention even after unprotected sex increased by 17 percent.
- "The number who knew there was something she could do and specified she could take birth control pills increased by 23 percent.
- "Of the number who knew there was something she could do, 20 percent said they learned about it on ER."

They commented, "With 34 million people watching this episode, it is possible that five to six million people learned about emergency contraception for the first time on this show." This is positive power!

"The increased awareness did not last," the report continues. "While immediately after the episode 67 percent of the viewers knew that a woman has options, only 50 percent retained that awareness two and a half months later. That's pretty good motivation, not only for incorporating healthy, safer sex methods into TV programming, but for being sure the message is *repeated* for longer term retention."

Because the heroes in our culture today are the celebrities, it is even more important that their messages or messages about them in the media be responsible. Cindy Crawford, the popular model, made a start with her TV program, "Sex with Cindy Crawford."[5] It was a program of substance and interest in spite of the titillating title.

In one episode, Crawford interviewed teens who write and edit *Sex, Etc., A Newsletter by Teens for Teens.* This newsletter is written by teens of high school age, and published by the Network for Family Life Education in New Jersey. The young people were honest with Crawford. They told her about the debate over the possible distribution of condoms in school. They discussed their own attitudes about sex.

Crawford also spoke with therapists and others about teen sexuality, and reported on the Kaiser Family Foundation findings that three out of five teens believe the information they get about sex and birth control comes too late.

ABC-TV captured the audience by using Cindy Crawford to host, and it kept the audience by having short interviews with interesting topics. It varied the message throughout, using teaching tactics effective teachers use in classrooms. The attention span of students, and of both young and older listeners, is short unless their attention is captured. The media know this better than anyone, but when they capture that attention, their opportunities to educate are limitless.

Can Media Make a Difference?

Positive messages from the media make a difference. Oprah names a book title and book sales skyrocket. In *The Media and the Message,*[6] published by the National Campaign to Prevent Teen Pregnancy, the authors document the media campaign for the "designated driver." They describe the public service announcements, messages embedded into regular programming, and the celebrities engaged to deliver a powerful and consistent message about the dangers of drinking and driving.

The results? Increased use of the designated driver, fewer fatalities, stigmatization of drinking and driving. The proof that it worked? The term "designated driver" became part of our everyday vocabulary, even appearing in the latest dictionaries. The format for a successful "Safer Sex or No Sex" campaign is here.

The Stanford Three Community Study describes a campaign urging citizens to get physically fit. A media blitz produced a 15 to 20 percent decrease in heart attack risk compared with a similar community that did not have the media campaign and in which risk increased.

An interesting corollary of this study is that another community, in which the media campaign was combined with face-to-face instruction in cardiovascular risk reduction skills, showed even greater levels of success.[7]

A "Felicity" episode on TV with a story line of date rape included a hotline. After the show the station received 800 calls from teens; a rerun of the same program got 500 calls. On two "Roseanne" TV programs, Roseanne indicated that she was using the birth control pill and her partner was using a condom. This normalized their use and encouraged millions of teens to think about birth control if they are going to have sex.[8]

Harness the Power

The United States needs to harness the power of television and other media to be a positive influence on teens, something Europe has been doing so successfully. Madison Avenue needs to work with young people to produce posters and TV ads that send the message "Safer Sex or No Sex." They need programming that incorporates the condom into sexual intercourse scenes, whether shown or implied.

Advocates for Youth in Washington, DC, is making a start. During a recent Let's Talk Month, they circulated colorful large posters showing a male and female, T-shirts and jeans back view, his arm around her waist, walking together, with the caption, "Gotcha keys? Gotcha cash? Gotcha condoms?"

If we were in the Netherlands, or France or Germany, this poster would be displayed everywhere, in high schools, theaters, drugstores, teen organizations, bus stops — any place a teen could see it and remind himself or herself to be prepared. In our country, the only place I saw the poster was the copy I received in the mail.

We can do the job we need to do, but we all have to go to

86   ***Safer Sex: The New Morality***

work. We have to agree on one clear message, make it consistent, make it persistent, and make it work. And of all of the players who influence teens, according to Barbara Huberman of Advocates for Youth, "The media are the most important. They could be not only the message, but also the messenger, the advocate, the mentor, the educator. They could become the most important force in the country for a turnaround in teen attitudes, teen health, and teen birth."

Let's add, not only a force for a turnaround in teen attitudes, but also for a turnaround in all of our attitudes, young and old alike.

The press must be desensitized to the allure of sex and sensitized to the fact that not all the public wants sex and scandal all of the time. There are people reading and watching who want substance over sound byte.

Advocates need to communicate that sex is about public health, not about politics, morality, money, or the cultural war. This is the job for the media. They need to reduce sexual fantasy in ads and programming, and initiate sexual normalcy and reality — the joys of committed sex and the dangers of unsafe sex. Truth in advertising has never been so important.

Participants in the European study tour were asked to make recommendations to our media about public education campaigns. Their list included:

- Media campaigns that focus on Safer Sex or No Sex.
- Government money to support the media.
- Cooperation between government and media.
- Cooperation between the media and public interest groups to produce clear messages with a public health focus.
- Projects that encourage producers to include positive health images.
- Heavy-duty holiday campaigns, which is the time when many teen pregnancies occur.
- Involvement of youth in the development of youth-targeted media campaigns.

Media's Sexual Script

Research tells us that not enough teens use contraception. What is the role of the media here? Kate Folb is the director of the Media Project of Advocates for Youth in Washington, DC. This organization works with the media to encourage them to keep adolescents in mind when producing their programming. Folb says that in the absence of enough parental conversation, inadequate sex education in the schools, and the conflicting advice from religious institutions, media provide most of the sexual scripts for teens. Shows are attractive, compelling, and exciting, and young people are watching and listening.

It's up to the public to teach the media. "Give them the script," said Jane Brown, University of North Carolina, Chapel Hill, speaking at the conference, "Messages and Methods for the New Millennium: A Round Table on Adolescents and Contraception" in February, 1999. "Since the media are the primary teachers of the sexual script, include the realities. Teach them how to talk about contraception, teach them the behavior that goes with being responsible. Incorporate healthy sexual messages with the passion. In fact, make it sexy to use condoms." The television writers told Brown that condoms destroy the mood. Brown replied that as the most creative people in the country, the writers should be able to figure it out.

The media may want to make the necessary changes, if for no other reason, out of self-interest. Rebecca W. Rimel, of the Pew Charitable Trust,[9] writes, "As we move toward a new century, the erosion of trust in the media has become as big a story as some of the scandals they cover. Can our society solve its problems if the public turns away from Congress, the Presidency, and the media?" She points out that the press doesn't tell society what to think but that it does frame the message and the way it is delivered. Most of all, it decides what to include and what to exclude. She is talking about news but the problem is the same for entertainment.

Kathleen Hall Jamieson, dean of the Annenberg School for Communication, University of Pennsylvania, gives us hope. She says, "It doesn't take that many people to get the system to change. Talk back to the media," she says. "Agitate for change."[10] She is talking about news coverage, the sound bytes that reporters think the public wants. But the public wants real information, too, just as it wants healthy messages about sex delivered to all the public, not only to teens.

The Media Project's work is paying off. Kate Folb reports that the SHINE Awards this year prove that the industry is finally "getting it." SHINE (Sexual Health in Entertainment) honors popular teen programs for incorporating sexual responsibility into their programming.

Programs honored in 1999 included "Felicity," "Moesha," and "Party of Five" TV shows. Felicity and Moesha each decide she's ready to have sex, wants to be prepared, and goes to the clinic to learn about birth control. "Party of Five" received the award for a sequence of episodes dealing with effective communication about sex between Claudia (the little sister) and Sarah (Bailey's girlfriend who is in her late teens). The persistence and support of this arm of Advocates for Youth are bringing about change.

Parents, mentors, and concerned citizens can lobby for media responsibility. Parents can monitor what their children see and hear at home and be there for them when they are exposed to excesses. We can all model respect and responsibility by our behavior. We *can* make a difference.

In the long run, we can't blame the media, the advertisers, the scriptwriters, or the producers. We can blame only ourselves. If we don't let the media know our convictions, if we don't inform them of our unhappiness with their lack of responsibility, if we don't offer our support in producing responsible programming for teens, if we don't boycott programs and products that show no respect to our children, then we get what they give us.

Unless we put our efforts behind our concerns, our love/hate affair with the media ends up being a love/hate affair with ourselves.

5

Evolving Role of Religion

Quite frankly, in our Baptist life the idea is you don't participate in sexual relations until you are married, period. But that is an exaggeration of the responsibility part and ignores the reality that experimentation is going to take place. So you need some methods, you need some tools for them to fall back on. I see that balance there, the both/and, and that's where I am.

Reverend Frank Hawkins, Tennessee

Is there anything that brings out the best and the worst in people, the most loving and the most aggressive feelings, the most passionate and the most lethargic expressions of attitude, the most peaceful and the most warlike behaviors as does religion? My mother used to advise me against arguing about religion with strangers. "You can only get into trouble," she said. Good advice. I think she might have added, "or with friends." I have seen good friends get so heated in a discussion of religion that they have to tiptoe back into their friendship.

Religion causes so much intensity of feeling because it touches our most basic values, our most basic beliefs, our most basic anxieties about our lives and how we live them, and even how we die them.

Religion involves ethics, morality, right and wrong, justice and mercy, good and bad. These are the rules by which we conduct ourselves. The codes by which we raise our children. The commandments by which we care for our elderly. The religious or secular laws by which we judge the rightness or wrongness of giving or taking birth and death. These concepts guide our ways, touch upon our most basic fears, and serve us well or serve us badly. Why wouldn't they cause passionate debate? If we have a belief system and it's working for us, why wouldn't we question another system that we either don't know or don't believe in?

Why did the Crusaders put heads of babies on spikes if not in the name of religion? Why do some religious fundamentalists today kill doctors who provide abortion if not in the name of religion?

Jehovah's Witnesses insist that only they will be saved during Armageddon because this is what they truly believe. Why would they work so diligently to convert others if they did not think it true?

Why does the Islamic Taliban forbid women to work outside their homes and force them to hide from male eyes? They believe they are following the will of their god.

Why would ultra-Orthodox Jews throw stones at groups of Reform and Conservative Jews praying at the Western Wall in Jerusalem? They believe that only their form of Judaism is valid.

Why did Christian missionaries in Hawaii cover the nakedness and force Christianity on Hawaiians who were living in simplicity and naturalness? They believed they were inspired by their god to do so.

All these things and more have been done in the name of religion. All believed that they were right and doing God's work on earth.

Ethics and Beliefs

Ethics are at the root of religious beliefs. When duties conflict, the believer is faced with a moral dilemma. Which is the greater right, the greater wrong? These are not easy questions to answer.

The ethical philosophers who guided our cultures during the last three hundred years included, among others, Locke, Rousseau, Bentham, Kant and Mill. They realized that ethnic groups, classes, and religions needed some type of common ethic that each could embrace in the resolution of their disagreements. Each of these great thinkers gave us a type of ethical code by which to guide ourselves.

We may not even be aware of the religious philosophy behind our value systems, but we know what we believe. Most of us think we know what is right and what is wrong. For some, based on religious teachings, an act is inherently right or wrong with no questions asked. For others, human beings can decide together whether an act is right or wrong. Still others believe an act is right if it brings happiness to the most people. And others guide their lives through their own consciences, believing goodness does not depend on religious beliefs.

For those who believe that there is only one right way, all other moral or religious codes are wrong. The more fundamentalist the believers, the more they believe in the literal interpretation of their tenets. Herein lie the problems that surround abortion, contraception, sexuality education, duty and obligation, the benefits to society, and individual rights and responsibilities.

Many of us are guided by the ethical code that there are universal "goods" that could benefit both society and individuals. There are rights and responsibilities that all could incorporate into their world views, and legal rights could back up the moral rights.

Countries in Europe, choosing the health and well-being of their youth as the basis for decision making, agreed to universals by which to guide their education, their media campaigns, and their governmental decision making. The reproductive health and well-being of their citizens, principally their adolescents, became the goal, and all rallied around it. What was good for society became good for each of the citizens, as teen pregnancy and birth rates fell, as sexually transmitted infection rates fell, and as abortion rates fell.

Those who objected to abortion were pleased; those whose public health issues around sexually transmitted infections were paramount were happy; and those who worried about too early parenting were satisfied.

That these outcomes entailed comprehensive sexuality education on the part of schools and the media became less important than that the society as a whole was benefiting from the ethics of "do unto others as you would have others do unto you." Respect for children was returned with respect by children; expecting responsibility from children elicited responsibility from them.

Positive/Negative Influence of Religion

What does religion offer that draws so many people to it? At its best it offers answers, a connectedness, belief in something other than oneself, a sense of history, stories, rituals, shared experience, drama, music, song, oneness and togetherness. It provides an opportunity for fervor, a focus, structure, a support system, a sense of community, and friendship. It cultivates a sense of spirituality that enhances inner peace.

Nanette Dizney, program director of a school for pregnant and parenting teens in Bradenton, Florida, found that the church was her support system when her husband left her with four children. Not only did she find guidance there for her teenagers, she found role models and mentors in fellow church members and in the clergy. The church supplied far more than religious training as her children became involved in social, musical, and athletic activities.

Parents for whom religion is working find that the church helps them guide their children; their children find like-minded peers; the education establishes moral codes and behaviors that their friends follow so the peer pressure is positive. For Nanette and her children, the church was a savior. This is religion and the church at their best.

Young people benefit from a loving, caring religion with its rituals, traditions, and structure. But should it stop there? What about socialization, goals, and the difficulties of transition from child status to adolescent status? Surely religion could be a positive influence here. When it chooses to address only one of these issues, whether teens should indulge in sexual experimentation, and the answer is a flat "No sex — abstinence only," it misses out.

Like any other influence in young people's lives, religion can play a very positive role or it can play a very negative one. A loving god can model love, caring and safety; an angry god can model punishment, guilt, and fear. Religion can provide a powerful role model for young people, a safety net within which to learn socialization, leadership, followership, respect, and responsibility. Its role should not be intimidation. Yet, like any other place where power is too heavily invested in one person or a small group, there is the opportunity for abuse.

Inflexibility of Fundamentalism

Fundamentalism in any form is by the nature of its inflexibility, intimidating. When the rules are infallible, and the Book is the answer, rules shall not be broken and therefore must be enforced when they are.

The big problems arise with those who believe in the *either/or* rather than the *both/and.* Those who believe that the only truths are from the word of god and guide their lives by those words limit their lives and their families' lives. It doesn't matter which Book we are talking about; the issue is that if it's not in the Book, then it's not good, not right, not allowed. It's either right or it's wrong.

This narrowness of vision makes for a narrowness of life for the believers. But, in a democracy like ours, it's their choice. Those who believe differently do not take issue with this. It is when people seek to force their values and their ideas of right and wrong on others that many of us object. If they then exert political pressure by lobbying with politicians and supporting them financially so that the laws of the land will reflect their religious views, then we really object.

The half billion dollars of federal and state funding for Abstinence Only education is an example of such influence. (See chapter 7.) Once we are into the realm of the political, with religion and politics arm in arm, then our constitutional rights and our human rights are in jeopardy. As one 13-year-old eighth grader said, "Just because you really believe something, it doesn't give you the right to decide for everybody else."

Broadening Religious Education

Too controlling or too distant approaches are both missed opportunities for healthy teen growth and development. With no exploration of the issues of curiosity, hormones, drives, and the powerful influence of irresponsible, sexually driven media in these most vulnerable years, religion loses its opportunity to teach about love, commitment, respect, and the pairing of sex with momentous life issues.

With instruction that includes teen interaction, discussion, and peer involvement, the data inform us that "religious faith and a strong moral sense play vital roles in protecting teen boys and girls from too-early sexual activity and teen pregnancy."[1]

Changes in Role of Religion

Religious leaders have long known that their institutions can play a unique role in supporting sexuality education in their community. In 1968 the National Council of Churches Commission on Marriage and Family, the Synagogue Council

of America Committee on Family, and the United States
Catholic Conference Family Life Bureau joined together to
write an "Interfaith Statement on Sex Education."[2]

Thirty years later, May, 1999, twenty theologians from
diverse denominations joined together to write "The Religious Declaration on Sexual Morality, Justice, and Healing."
As of March 14, 2000, the declaration had received 1,526
endorsements. The role of the church had broadened and there
was an outpouring of support for the change.

Debra W. Haffner, president of SIECUS (Sex Information
and Education Council of the United States), says religious
institutions must become involved in sexuality education.
They are in a unique position because they reach so many
people, especially youth. Sexuality is the source of much
alienation and hurt to many Americans, and faith communities could help them heal. Moreover, young people say they
want their religious institution to do more. The opportunity
is there.[3]

Two ministers I interviewed, one from Tennessee and one
from Maine, were raised fundamentalist. Both were also
exposed to more liberal points of view as young people, and
both have developed broader philosophies as they have
worked with their constituencies. They shared what they
thought the role of religion should or could be relative to
sexuality. The Reverend Frank Hawkins, a 60-year old Baptist
minister whose quote begins this chapter, said:

*My basic thought on sexuality is that it is good. I think the
underlying message that we need to get across to people,
whether they are the radical right or the radical left, is that
it's good, that it's a gift. Along with the gift, just like the gift
of freedom, it has to be balanced with the dynamic of
responsibility.*

*There is no way to avoid experimentation with our sexual-
ity. If you put young people in a straight jacket, their sexuality
will cry out and will take forms that will be irresponsible. The
experimentation needs to be a delicate dance between parents
and teenagers. Teens' freedom should be respected, and*

*parents need to keep in touch, but at a safe distance.
Teenagers can have their secrets, and those secrets are
respected, as long as the young people know that they can
talk with their parents but don't have to. Then they are
developing their individuality.*

*The extreme right views truth and reality only in terms
of either/or logic, you either agree with them or you are
wrong . . . and the extreme left probably has the flaw of not
understanding the responsibility part along with the freedom.
So it's that balance between responsibility and freedom, trying
to find a way to help young people balance these two. A
comprehensive approach is needed because most truths are
both/and. Many people feel we came too far in the sixties, and
now there has been the reaction.*

*Quite frankly, in our Baptist life the idea is you don't
participate in sexual relations until you are married, period.
But that is an exaggeration of the responsibility part and
ignores the reality that experimentation is going to take place.
So you need some methods, you need some tools for them to
fall back on. I see that balance there, the both/and, and that's
where I am.*

*The Catholic religion is very strong on parenting, and they
see human sexuality as existing for parenting almost exclu-
sively. The theology is you participate in sex to have children.
When it comes to practicality, however, many Catholics don't
adhere to that. They practice birth control.*

*In the Protestant tradition there is the motif of the destruc-
tion of aloneness, Adam and Eve coming together to destroy
aloneness. This was not just for Adam, but for Eve also. She
was not a second thought in the mind of God. It is not Eve's
position just to serve man, to gratify him and produce babies
for him. Their companionship is basic.*

*Sexuality is for the destruction of aloneness and for the
creation of community between two people. When that occurs
there is always the possibility of children . . . where there is
love and respect between two people, and affirmation,
where one is not being used by the other, then you have a*

relationship that is worthy of parenthood. Sexuality is not a choice; it is part of our nature and we must use it responsibly.

The Reverend Douglas W. Drown, Bingham, Maine, is a 48-year-old Congregational minister who considers himself a reformed fundamentalist:

When I was young my pastor was a fundamentalist and a good Bible teacher, but even at that age I didn't agree with everything he had to say. I was a little uncomfortable with the rigidity of fundamentalism. I tried to escape from it. I had a friend who was a Unitarian minister at the other end of the spectrum from my church. At high school I was asked to join the choir at his church. He was a humanist, a very interesting fellow who began to broaden my understanding of things spiritual. I think this was the beginning of the tempering of my boyhood fundamentalism.

In time I came to realize that people are more important than ideology, more important than trying to promulgate a dogmatic view on spirituality and life in general. With fundamentalists everything is black or white. There is a Biblical answer to every question, but there are a lot of areas in life that are very grey. I found that to be true early on in the ministry.

A woman who came to me some years ago was hurting because she was experiencing a lot of unhappiness in her marriage. She had aspirations in life that her husband disagreed with. They were both fundamentalists. He had abandoned Catholic conservatism and exchanged one kind of rigidity for another. He was verbally abusive to her. Her pastor told her it was her problem, that the Bible says a woman should submit to her husband. If she did this she would not be unhappy.

I told her the problem lay with her husband. The best thing she could do was get out of the relationship, at least temporarily. I was young at the time and it was a hard thing for me to do, but I saw her real need.

Do these ministers, one in conservative Tennessee and the

other in liberal Maine, presage change within churches? As we see more pressure being brought to bear by the religious right, are we also seeing change toward more liberal points of view? James F. Clarity reports from Dublin that as times change in Ireland so does the influence of the Roman Catholic Church. As Ireland becomes richer it also becomes less formally religious, much like the rest of Europe. He says, "The church (is) searching for a new role, something more akin to spiritual adviser than rigid arbiter of social and sexual mores. The Church bishops now talk more about individual conscience on matters of abortion or divorce, rather than about mortal sin or eternal damnation. Condoms are widely available."[4]

In Mexico, another bastion of Catholicism, there has been a reduction in fertility rates as the children of large families realize that "small families live better."[5] There has been a drop from seven children per woman in 1965 to 2.5 per woman today. Because of demographics and economics, Mexico is in the midst of a shift from governmental and church support for large families to support for smaller families.

Over-population and the scarcity of jobs that result in so many Mexicans coming to the United States are a major influence in the new thinking. Family planning services have proliferated, and the average Mexican is also exposed to lifestyles of people all over the world through the internet, television, and other media. Church influence has waned under these conditions, and many families are practicing birth control.

Positive signs of social change are also beginning to appear within religious denominations in attitudes. The emerging acceptance of homosexuality is an example. In June of 1999 sixty-eight Methodist ministers jointly blessed a union between two women church members, causing church leaders to charge the ministers with violating church law.[6] The real story is that sixty-eight ministers were willing to jeopardize their careers in support of their belief that homosexuals were entitled to the same privileges of the church as heterosexuals.

The Central Conference of American Rabbis approved a resolution to sanction same-sex unions, offering the protection of Reform Judaism to clergy who officiate. This is the first major religious denomination to affirm gay and lesbian unions.[7]

The role of religion can extend beyond its own doors and its own constituencies. On June 18, 1999, a pre-dawn arson attack on three Sacramento, California, Jewish synagogues caused nearly $1 million in damages.[8] The congregations, shocked and fearing a rise of anti-Semitism in their community, flocked to a Friday night service to express their support of their Temples and leadership. They were surprised and thrilled to find 1800 people from all over the community, including African Americans, Caucasians, Asians, members of nearly every Protestant Church, Catholics, Buddhists, and Hare Krishnas coming to show their support.

Northern California United Methodist leaders who were attending a conference in Sacramento donated $6,000 to replace library books destroyed in the fire. Even the most suspicious Jews in the congregation, who couldn't believe that Christians could be so kind to Jews, had tears in their eyes. Here's a role religion can play — standing up to anti-anyone, supporting fellow humans in word and deed, and helping to remove the fears and stigma of differentness.

Areas of Agreement

Perhaps we could come to a meeting of the minds about the importance of religion. Even those who choose to believe in no religion will usually recognize that it serves an important function for millions of people in the world. Recent research indicates that of the 48 percent of 15- to 19-year-olds who said they were virgins, "nearly one-half said that the main reason they had abstained from sex was that it was against their religion or morals."[9] We could encourage respect for all beliefs, or for none, thus eliminating the pressure that one group would seek to place on another.

We might come to agreement that the *values* of religionists and the values of humanists are not so different. Those who do not attend a house of worship may still believe very strongly in the tenets of the Ten Commandments. And those who do worship regularly may not live their beliefs in their everyday lives. One does not necessarily equate with the other.

People of good faith, whether that faith is God-centered or not, can ally with one another behind the *both/and* banner. We must agree on the goal that combines both religious and secular morality — the physical, emotional, and mental health of our young people. To achieve that goal we must as a society agree to educate everyone about:

- The beauty and joy of sex in a quality relationship.
- The disrespect of unsafe sex.
- The dangers of HIV/AIDS and other sexually transmitted infections (STIs).
- The benefits of delaying sexual intercourse.
- The inhumanity of having unwanted children.
- The irresponsibility of having abortions that could have been prevented by protected sex.

This would entail dialogue with federal and local government, the media, the schools, parent groups, religious groups, and non-governmental agencies.

Involving Religious Leaders

The religious fundamentalists, who are over-sensitized to sex and its implications, need to be desensitized. They might learn to see that it's not all bad, that it's not all fantasy, that it's not immoral. Then there are the ultra liberals who understand that sex is a normal part of the human condition, and don't understand why everyone doesn't agree with them. They must be sensitized to the fears of the religious right.

They need to be able to address these individuals' anxieties and dislike their views without disliking the people. Each must learn to communicate with those who have a different point of view.

What else can religious leaders do? First, they can examine their morality base. If it's an *either/or* model, they can agree to stop, look, and listen to other points of view. They can survey their congregants to find out where they are in terms of comprehensive sexuality education that recommends abstinence as the first and best protection, and teaches contraception and disease prevention methods as well as communication skills and respect between partners.

They can talk with other religious leaders to learn how they deal with sexuality education for their teens. They can examine and implement the sexuality curricula developed by their own denominations. They can observe sexuality education classes in their local school districts and talk with the educators there. They can talk with their own teens.

They can share the data gathered in the 1999 SIECUS and Advocates for Yourth report that show overwhelmingly that adults want their children to be offered comprehensive sexuality education in their schools. (See page 123).[10]

The Advocacy Manual for Sexuality Education, Health and Justice: Resources for Communities of Faith[11] offers guidance for religious group leaders. To address the needs of teens, they recommend helping young people understand what their faith says about love and sexuality, and reaching out to other communities that work with young people.

The Role of Religion

Dr. Jany Rademakers, Research Coordinator at NISSO (Netherlands Institute for Social Sexological Research), stated that religion was important in her country in the fifties. People were accepting of the notion of abstinence until marriage and averse to contraception and abortion. But the sixties changed it all as solidarity, feminism, the pill, the legality of abortion, and the power of students brought about a societal change. People became less accepting of church doctrine, and the control of religion on their lives diminished.

Our country may be ready now. Perhaps we will see a diminishing of fundamentalist church influence on sexuality in the new century. Hopefully, the churches will begin to play a greater role in a responsible approach to healthy communities and support of young people.

The Reverend David E. Richards suggests a way to restore dialogue that has been terminated. He says, "One way . . . is to move the discussion from rules to values. It is possible that if some agreement can be achieved in regard to the values of sexual health, it may be easier to discuss the 'rules' of sexual health."[12]

I propose that religion could not only catch up but could become a leader in the acceptance of a new sexual morality:

Thou shalt view sexuality as healthy and natural,
and express it wisely.
Thou shalt not have unsafe sex.
Thou shalt not give or get a sexually transmitted disease.
Thou shalt not use abortion as a contraceptive device.
Thou shalt not give birth to unwanted, unplanned children.
Thou shalt show respect for and take responsibility for
thine own body
and that of thy partner.

When religion becomes a partner with teens, parents, schools, business, government, and the media in spreading the word of "Safer Sex or No Sex," our young people, and all of society, will benefit. Religious congregations might also benefit as young people decide to look into the youth groups and activities, and who knows? *They might even get involved in their faith community.*

CHAPTER
6

Sexuality Education Is Everywhere

In fifth grade guys would ask, "Are you a virgin?" and I'd answer, "No." I thought it was a bad word because I didn't know what it meant.

When someone older talks about something you don't know, you tell them you know all about it so you won't be embarrassed. They want to be cool so they tell you anyhow, and sometimes you end up learning something after all.

Alissa, 15

We view teen sexual behavior in the United States through a number of lenses: It's a private family matter. It's a public health issue. It's a moral failing. It's a political issue. What we often don't understand is that it is a developmental issue for young people. This often causes confusion in our sexuality education efforts.

Informal Sexuality Education

When we think about sexuality education, many of us picture a teacher and students in a school classroom. But formal teaching is not the only avenue for student learning. Young people get informal sexuality education every day of their lives. They learn about sex just as they learn about eating, dressing, and interacting with others. They learn from what we tell them and what we don't tell them, from what we do and don't do. They learn from our reactions to sexual situations, and from our attitudes about our own sexuality and that of others. They learn from TV, radio, magazines, movies, newspapers, and each other.

A child who has been sexually abused has had a lesson about sexual violence and its effects. A child who has observed two caring adults relating to each other has had a lesson about the bonds of an intimate relationship. Children learn from the moment they are born and are put into the arms of a loving or indifferent caretaker.

Most parents, whether comfortable about it or not, realize they play a role as sexuality educators for their children. Other people that children see, however, may have no idea that they are also sexuality educators. From the first nurse who handles a newborn to the preschool teacher, the school librarian, the writer for TV, and the morning disc jockey, all are teaching about sex whether or not they are aware of their role.

Store clerks teach lessons as well. As I research and write this book I am always looking for condom machines and condom displays. How easy or how difficult is it for young people to find them? Recently I went to the local drugstore in a small town. I noticed the aisle sign that listed "Condoms, Large Size Soap Powders, Bleaches." I found every type of soap powder and bleach imaginable, but not a single condom. When I asked the cashier at the checkout counter to help me, she said, "Oh, we just moved them to another aisle where we had a lot more room. They're at the end of the aisle with the women's sanitary pads."

"In that section," I asked, "would a young boy find them?"

"Oh, yes," she said, "they do. And I never tease them when they check them out."

"What do you mean?" I asked.

"Well, some of the cashiers tease them and say things like, 'I know what you're going to do,' but I always say, 'Good for you, you're being careful'." She smiled, pleased with herself.

Is this sexuality education? Of course. Both the placement and the response to his purchase give the teen male a message. If he finds the condoms at all, he notices that someone may comment on them. Nobody, noticing the film he bought, says, "I know what you're going to do." A teen buying a condom may elicit a comment, whether it's to tease or to praise. The female teen, while she may find the condoms more easily, is no doubt exposed to the same kind of commentary.

What have these teens learned? It's not comfortable to buy condoms. Maybe they'd be better off to forget about them and take a chance with unprotected sex. We're a long way from building safer sex for young people into our society.

Other Approaches to Sexuality Education

Contrast our American approach with these two accounts of sexuality education. Bart, now 30, grew up in the Netherlands. Mel, his fiancée, now 25, grew up in England.

Bart: *When I was young my father was a psychologist so he always took us along to university classes and we were tested for everything as you can imagine. I was getting involved in sex education at about three or four. He told me it was the normal thing that goes around in the world, nothing to be ashamed of. People love each other, hug each other, have sex together, but the thing is you have to be careful of your actions. You have to be careful and be responsible for yourself. You get used to seeing people kiss each other. When I was getting older, about 7 years old, they gave us early education about sexuality in school. They used all the real words, you know, no nonsense about it. This is it, just the way they would teach adults, which made it really interesting. Since I already knew about it from my parents, I got to know what sex was all about, positions and everything.*

"Were the kids comfortable with this?"

Bart: *The way it was taught was comfortable. I could notice the teachers were watching reactions. They tried to bring out issues and get the kids to speak about it. They asked us if we saw parents kissing and hugging and asked how we felt about that.*

"Did you get into feelings, drives, hormones in England?" I asked Mel.

Mel: *No. The English are very reserved about that.*

Bart: *In Holland they really get into the whole thing, even with little kids. They said, "Oh, yes, if you are a female or a male it is very different. If you're female, you will mature faster, and be more interested in boys. For the boys it happens later on. When they get a low voice and everything starts to grow they get more interested and become more attracted to girls." What they talk about is this feeling, this urge, but still not knowing what is going on. They let us talk about that. They say you won't know what is going on, and they try to explain what is going to happen.*

"Did this help you?"

Bart: *Oh, yes, I knew what to expect and I was getting ready to think about girls, not that I was really into it. I still preferred sports and boy activities.*

"Contraception? Did they teach it? Did they show you how to use condoms?"

Bart: *Oh, yes, the Double Dutch method, using both a female birth control method and condoms for diseases. They taught us how to put a condom on, about the pill, too, and how many times you have to take it. They taught about the coil (IUD), how the doctor puts it in, what to do if you get pregnant, and the morning after pill. Say you start fooling around, no excuse at all, and have sex unprotected. If so, they tell you what to do. They really are into that. What to do, who to tell, where to go, boys and girls go together. It's the responsibility of both.*

"Mel? Did you hear that in England?"

Mel: *No, I don't think we ever really talked about being pregnant. Just conventional sex ed.*

Bart: *They also talked about abortion. First you have to tell* *your parents, although it depends on what age you are. If you're old enough to take care of your own body, you can do it yourself. If you're young, you have to tell your parents because they have to pay. The kids couldn't pay, so you have to tell your parents. They take you to the doctor who sends you to the specialist and you get the abortion. It's the prudent thing to do.*

"Did you have media campaigns?"

Mel: *With all the AIDS scare they showed the shock of it basically, and they were convincing. Some of them were just about using condoms and they had this wire fence. They started with a boy on one side and a girl on the other, holding hands, just to show the relationship.*

You could see what was going to happen after. No condom. And then it said to use a condom, but didn't show it. Then after the scene ended, they showed the condom. Still restrained, very English.

Bart: *In Holland we show posters, magazines, heterosexuals, homosexuals, biracial, funny ones, jokes that are really serious. You see three shots of couples, a boy and girl, two boys, and two girls. In the first scene the boy and girl are getting together, getting drunk, getting into a sex position. The girl pushes back, yells stop! and says not until you put this on. She takes the condom out of her jeans.*

Mel: *Ours showed scenes to let people know not to be embarrassed when buying condoms. One shows a boy asking, "Can I have a ccc . . . ccccc . . . ?" and finally the clerk says, "Oh you mean you want a condom!" and shouts it out. This was in England, about eight years ago.*

"Are these campaigns still going on?"

Bart: *Yes, in Holland.*

Mel: *Not in England as much. My first memory about sex is when my twin sister and I were about 3 or 4 years old, quite young, and my mum gave us a book that was basically on sex. I remember we read this book quite a lot with my mum. She was quite embarrassed about the whole thing.*

It was a good book because it showed exactly how it happened. There was a cross section of the body and you could see the penis entering the vagina and you could see the vagina. This was quite young to be talking about it.

"If your mother was embarrassed, why do you think she gave it to you at that age?"

Mel: *I don't know, she never talked about it, even now. Maybe she did that so she wouldn't have to talk to us.*

"But you studied and read it together?"

Mel: *Yes. Then I went to junior school at age 7 and we had sex ed lessons with a series of three videos about how animals mated and how chickens laid eggs. They tried to teach us a bit. But I knew more than that already, and I think everyone else in the class knew more, too.*

"Did they ever talk about feelings and about puberty, and how it feels?"

Mel: *No, it was all biological and physical. But we knew about feelings and used to play mummies and daddies at school.*

"When you were older, as adolescents, did you continue to have sex ed?"

Mel: *Yes, we had personal education lessons once a week for half an hour at school. It was on sex, drugs, alcohol. We were in an all girls school from 12 to 16. In those lessons they taught us about contraception, the condom, the coil, the cap, and the pill. We used to have biology as well. They didn't teach us how to put on a condom, not at all. We used to play with them and giggle.*

At that age, 14 and 15, no one in my school was really interested in having sex at all. We had no teen pregnancies that I knew of.

How different this is from our attitudes, even for Mel, whose education was far less open and less liberal than Bart's. What we are missing in our country is the European model, particularly that of the Netherlands. They say, "Teach them, talk with them, listen to them, and explain the biology, the physiology, and the psychology. Most of all teach them respect and responsibility." The open approach, the non-judgmentalism, raises children who, as Bart puts it, "blend into society" and grow up to become responsible citizens.

Our Youth Need Guidance

Jane E. Brody, in "Teenagers and Sex: Younger and More at Risk,"[1] suggests that millions of American children are at risk for having unsafe sex. They need to learn how to resist pressures to have sex at young ages. They need to know how to protect themselves from unwanted consequences if they do have sexual intercourse. She cites the recent decline in the teen birth rate, but continues to worry as she compares our statistics with the rest of the developed world.

Brody tells us, "The earlier the sex, the greater the risk of contracting disease and the greater the risk of unwanted children. The data: Three million teens acquire an STI each year in the United States; one million teenage girls become pregnant, one half of them within the first six months of initial intercourse. With little instruction at home or at school on how to resist the pressures to have sex and with even more limited access to effective contraception, such consequences are hardly surprising."

Some education takes place at clinics operating throughout the country, many supported by the federally funded Title X. They provide young people with quality sexuality education as well as services for reproductive health. Planned Parenthood clinics are also a resource, and there are others built into youth programs, employment/job training, schools, and residential facilities for youth.

The depth of education offered at these clinics depends on the restrictions imposed by the community or the funding agency. A nurse at one clinic told me they weren't supposed to provide contraceptive information or contraceptives to children younger than 16, but she frequently looked the other way when she knew the young person was sexually active. "I felt it was my job to protect him or her from sexually transmitted infections as well as to protect the female from pregnancy. I just didn't ask for an age."

The Media Move On

Teenagers' infatuation with TV has spilled over to their love affair with the internet. It is the next frontier for sexuality education. We know of its popularity for pornographic sites.

Unfortunately, these reinforce the notions teens have gleaned from the media that sex has no consequences and is part of any relationship, no matter how young or how casual it is.

More good sexuality education on the internet would be a real plus for teens. The United Nations Population Fund Executive Director Nafis Sadik announced that her agency "is planning to offer sexuality education on the internet in its latest drive against population growth and AIDS."[2] This is good news for teens here as well as around the world.

In 1994 The Network for Family Life Education in New Jersey initiated a sexuality and health newsletter called *Sex, Etc., A Newsletter by Teens for Teens.*[3] Present distribution is 550,000 copies of each issue. It became so popular with schools,

Recommended Web Sites

- *Sex Etc., A Newsletter by Teens for Teens* — www.sxetc.org
- *Advocates for Youth* — www.advocatesforyouth.org
  Program and policy information about adolescent sexual health.
- *Annie E. Casey Foundation* — www.aecf.org
  Children and family health and well-being indicators.
- *Centers for Disease Control and Prevention (CDC)* —
  www.cdc.gov/nccdphp/divash.htm
  Youth risk behaviors, school and community health programs.
- *Child Trends, Inc.* — www.childtrends.org
  Analysis and statistics on a range of child and family issues.
- *National Campaign to Prevent Teen Pregnancy* —
  www.teenpregnancy.org
  Variety of data, information and resources on teen pregnancy.
- *Sexuality Information and Education Council of the U.S.* —
  www.siecus.org
  Parent, youth information, including surveys, publications.
- *Teenwire* — www.teenwire.com
  Discussions on personal, social and cultural youth topics.
- *The Alan Guttmacher Institute* — www.agi-usa.org
  Research and statistics on reproductive issues.
- *FOCUS on Young Adults* — http://www.pathfind.org/focus.htm
  Adolescent reproductive health issues worldwide.

churches, pregnancy prevention programs, clinics and others that in February, 1999, it launched a website (www.sxetc.org). With their teen slant, both the newsletter and the website offer insights into sex and other health issues truly relevant to teens' needs. See the box on the opposite page for additional web site addresses.

Interactive programs may be the best tool of all. Teens, familiar with video games, can use these skills to explore risks and consequences in the safe environment of a teen-friendly well-designed computer program.

Live teen theater is another source of sexuality education for young people. Theater-trained adult mentors work with young people to write and produce plays dealing with teen issues. Their themes include unplanned pregnancy, older men with younger girls, date rape, sexually transmitted infections, drugs, alcohol, and abuse. They present to groups in schools, theaters, and community gathering places. Their presentations stimulate important dialogue with their audiences. Their non-preaching, non-judgmental tone, that puts an emphasis on decision-making and healthy consequences, educates while it entertains.

Evolution of Sexuality Education

We've come a long way from the 1920s when Ula, now 88, was in a New Haven high school classroom of all girls. The boys, in their own classes, had science, but the girls had no science in their curriculum. She was a freshman at college when she had her first course in biology, Hygiene 101, and her first exposure to the workings of the human body. Up to then she knew nothing of reproduction.

But we still have a long way to go. We haven't come as far as Frederic's Swiss mother, who raised her sons in a tiny Swiss village of 150 people. Frederic, now forty years old, told me:

I remember vaguely that we did experiment sexually with our classmates when we were about seven or eight. We examined each other's bodies, both boys and girls. I remember a girl of the same age who wanted to stop in the forest on the way home and play doctor. Well, I told my mum what we did and asked her if that was all right. Yes, she said. That's OK. It's perfectly normal.

When we were a little older my mum said to my twin brother and me that now it was time we understood how babies are made and where they come from, and we don't talk about the stork anymore. "Now you're getting older and you really should understand what you're doing." She explained that there are different ways of enjoying sexual experiences and that you never want to do anything that would get a girl pregnant until you are married. But you can play and enjoy many things just like you have done already, and that's all part of sexual experience.

Are we confused by our attitudes about sex? Yes, most of us, not only teens. But, for teens, whose ability to make decisions is still in the formative stage, it's more serious. They need positive role modeling to help them.

We make the assumption that adults have already formed their value systems and are less influenced by irresponsible sex-driven messages. Nevertheless, the unplanned pregnancy rate is more than 50 percent among *adults*,[4] and the rates of dissemination of sexually transmitted infections are just as high for adults as for teens. Maybe we make a false assumption when we think that adults already know what's good for them. Perhaps we can all use a healthy dose of sexuality education.

It's time to stop being hypocritical and it's time to stop being hypercritical. We need to be just plain critical. We need to look carefully at our own attitudes and at the way we pass those attitudes on to our children. We need to be aware of the curricula that are being taught to our children in schools and to support those that are realistic and reach children in real ways.

We also need to become a force in our communities. The overriding goals of wholesome sexuality education are that young people learn the lessons of responsibility and respect for themselves and for their sexual partners.

Adults have no control over what children learn on their own. That's why parents and other caring mentors need to be "askable." Young people must feel safe about coming to them for answers. *Adults who can discuss conception and contraception without embarrassment and without judgment are the best teachers of all.*

7

Abstinence Only vs. Abstinence Plus

*We have to teach young kids under 15 about sex, how
not to get pregnant, how it's better not to have sex at all.
Guys pretend to love you but when they find out you're
pregnant they leave you. Sometimes your parents aren't
there for you, either.*

*When you're too young it's too hard, too much stress,
and too difficult to be good to a child when you don't have
the support and comfort you need for yourself. I learned
about contraception in the tenth grade, five years too late
for me.*

Cyndi, 19-year-old mother

Our culture is conflicted about asking the schools to communicate with our teens about sex. It's not sure what message
parents should be giving their young people at home. What is
appropriate for congregations and youth-serving organizations?

There is insecurity about how best to prepare youth to reach adulthood safe and comfortable with their sexuality.

The chart on pages 116-117 compares the European (Netherlands, France, Germany) sexuality education model with the two principal American models, Comprehensive including abstinence (A+) and Abstinence Only (AO).

There are many similarities between the European Approach to sexuality education and the United States Comprehensive model. They are both based on research. Each recognizes that young people are sexual human beings. Each teaches in an open, honest manner, encouraging teens to question. Each provides abstinence education as well as all other methods of contraception. Responsibility, respect, communication skills, and acceptance of personal beliefs are values. Each supports informed teen decision-making.

The basic difference between them is rooted in the cultures of the countries on the opposite sides of the Atlantic. While both support teen decisions about whether to remain abstinent or to become sexually active, the Europeans accept teen intercourse as part of intimate relationships. The American model, while its goals include teaching skills to enable teens to make responsible decisions, encourages delay. Europe stresses protection; America stresses delay.

The United States Abstinence models (Abstinence Only and Abstinence Until Marriage) are different from both of the above. They stress abstinence either until after high school graduation or until marriage. Obedience, chastity, and conformity are values.

The biggest difference between the American Comprehensive model and the European model is the support system that surrounds each one. In Europe the government, the media, the parents, and the community support the schools and reflect their values.

In the United States a Comprehensive program frequently is at odds with the local controlling organizations, i.e., school board, organized religion, citizen groups, city council, etc. No matter how comprehensive the education, if the surrounding community does not have the same values, the healthy sexuality education message is diluted and young people are confused.

Abstinence Only (AO)

Those who believe that only abstinence until marriage is appropriate base their concept of sexuality education on this premise. "Here are the moral and health-related reasons to be abstinent," students are told. "Now live your life according to this precept." No other type of sexuality education is needed, nor permitted.

Infection prevention and contraception are not considered except to suggest, contrary to research, that condoms and contraceptives don't work. Abstinence Only education is the answer, they say. It is interesting that the groups who opposed sexuality education in the schools in the 1960s are the ones leading the charge for abstinence until marriage in schools of today.

The United States Congress had enough support for this point of view in 1996 to make Abstinence Only education part of its Welfare Reform Act.[1]

Abstinence Plus Contraception (A+)

If we believe that Abstinence Only does not work for all teens, then we must provide Comprehensive Sexuality Education (A+). We begin with abstinence as the first and safest method of contraception. As we help students develop their understanding of contraception, we stress the importance of safer sex or no sex.

We teach negotiation skills with partners so that risks are reduced. We expose teens to information and services that are available to keep them from getting pregnant and from contracting sexually transmitted infections. We adopt a non-judgmental attitude, but we do not shy away from the seriousness of teen pregnancy and infection. We are honest. This is Abstinence Plus education. More than eight out of every ten Americans believe young people should be given information to protect themselves from unplanned pregnancies and STIs, in addition to information about abstinence.[2]

COMPARING SEXUALITY EDUCATION	
	Europe
	European Approach
I. Goal	Ensure all sexually active have necessary skills to behave responsibly.
II. Values **A. Responsibility**	Individual ethical behavior in choosing sexual health and responsibility.
B. Openness	Families, educators and healthcare providers have open, honest, consistent discussions with teens about sexuality. No subject taboo.
C. Morality	Individual ethic includes responsibility, love, respect, tolerance, equity.
D. Abstinence	Parents support both abstinent and sexually active teens in making responsible decisions.
III. Adult **Attitude**	Sexuality is a developmental and public health issue; no fear or shame. Accepting of teen sexual intercourse as part of intimate relationships. Youth valued, trusted.
IV. Sexuality **Education Model**	Encourage specific healthy behaviors. Young people initiate questions.
V. Government **Involvement**	Funds media campaigns, sexuality education in schools, clinics, national healthcare.
VI. Access to **Services**	Free and convenient availability of contraception, emergency contraception, counseling, abortion.
VII. Policy Basis	Research informs education.
VIII. Scope	K-12 specific education as well as in all curriculum.

COMPARING SEXUALITY EDUCATION	
United States	
Comprehensive Including Abstinence (A+)	**Abstinence Only (AO)** (Abstinence Until Marriage)
Promote sexual health, acquire skills to make responsible decisions.	Instruct unmarried teens to abstain from sexual intercourse until marriage.
Exercise responsibility in sexual relationships, including abstinence.	Show responsibility by abstaining from sex until marriage.
Provide opportunity for young people to question, assess family values, and develop their own.	Provide no information regarding contraception other than abstaining. Controversial topics avoided.
People respect diversity of personal beliefs regarding sexuality.	Group ethic requires conformity to one standard.
Abstaining from sexual intercourse is most effective method of preventing unplanned pregnancy and STIs/HIV.	Abstaining from sexual intercourse is the only accepted method of preventing unplanned pregnancy and STIs/HIV.
Sexuality is a developmental and public health issue. All persons have the right to make responsible sexual choices. All children should be loved and cared for.	Unmarried sexual intercourse is a moral failing. Adults know what is best for children. Children should obey their elders.
Provide accurate information and skills to enable young people to exercise responsibility. Children are encouraged to discuss sexuality.	Provide impetus for young people to abstain from sexual intercourse until marriage. Children not encouraged to discuss sexuality.
Some government funding of clinics.	Funds Abstinence Only education in schools and other locations.
Promote access to information and healthcare services for young people involved in sexual relationships.	Young people should not be involved in sexual relationships and do not need access to information and services.
Research informs education.	Politics/religion influence education.
K-12, usually embedded in family life education.	Middle school through high school. Specific education.

Abstinence and the United States Congress

In spite of this difference in ideology, or perhaps because of it, we still have to deal with the issues confronting teens and the larger society today. The public overwhelmingly wants sexuality education in the schools. Congress, however, disregarding the popular support for comprehensive sexuality education by both professionals and lay people, overwhelmingly supported an Abstinence Only education approach.

In 1996 the United States Congress voted with its dollars, granting $250 million to states to teach students about abstinence with the explicit provision that no mention be made of any other type of contraception except to discuss the failure rates.[3]

With mandated state matching grants of $3 to every $4 in federal money, this comes to almost half a billion dollars over a five-year period. In addition, the last federal budget (1999) called for an increase in funds for AO education for the next two years.

The most troubling fact is that this Abstinence Only education must *exclude* other information on birth control and STI prevention. This is happening in an era when the spread of AIDS and other sexually transmitted infections continues and teen pregnancy rates are far too high. It seems completely irresponsible that Congress, which has the potential to be so influential in a public health campaign, prohibits accurate health education and protection for life itself.

The Federal Abstinence Only program wants students to accept abstinence until marriage. (The average age for first marriage is about 27 today.) The objectives include learning that abstinence is the only certain way to avoid out-of-wedlock pregnancy and STIs, and teaches that sexual activity outside of marriage is likely to have harmful psychological and physical effects.

Its stated goals are to reduce the amount of teen sex, to reduce the number of babies born to teens outside of marriage, and to reduce sexually transmitted infections. I don't question the goals: I do question the methods.

I also question the statement that sex outside of marriage is likely to have harmful psychological and physical effects. Certainly young teens having babies is often harmful for both the teens and the babies.

However, there surely are many healthy sexual relationships between unmarried older teens or adults that do not have harmful effects. The harmful effects are caused by a society that scorns teen sex, that is judgmental, that limits access to contraception, and that legislates ideological or religion-based programs backed with federal money.

The good news is that the Federal Abstinence Only legislation appropriated six million dollars for the purpose of evaluating these programs. Although not nearly enough, it is heartening that there will be some evaluation.

Up to now we have *no* validated, replicated research showing that Abstinence Only education makes a difference in teen sexual behavior. We do have such proof that Abstinence Plus (Comprehensive Sexuality Education) has lowered pregnancy rates across the country.

Where Do You Stand?

We're at the point now when most of us want to achieve the European *results* (very low teen birth rate, decreased abortion and HIV/AIDS rate). The great debate centers around Abstinence Only and Comprehensive Sexuality Education models. What type of sexuality education will work best?

To get the most out of this chapter, and to clarify your position on this issue, first take a simple quiz. No one but you will ever know your answers unless you choose to share them.

1. What year were you born?

2. How helpful to you was the sexuality education you received either at home, in school, or elsewhere?

3. If you were not abstinent until marriage, at what age did you first have voluntary vaginal sexual intercourse?

4. If married, were you sexually abstinent until then?

5. If you married, how old were you?

6. If you never married, have you remained sexually abstinent?

After you have taken the quiz, go back to the Introduction and read the personal histories over the decades of the twentieth century, especially the one that pertains to your teen era. Now read the ones that pertain to the teens of today.

Juggle all these ideas as you read and think about the cases that could be made for Abstinence Only *and* for Comprehensive Sexuality Education that includes abstinence and contraception (Abstinence Plus).

Abstinence Only and Abstinence Plus advocates can find some areas of agreement. They may agree that the media is infatuated with sex, and that it distorts sex and intimacy. They may also agree that parents play a vital role in helping teens delay sexual activity.

The two groups break ranks, however, when Abstinence Only advocates strongly question the safety of condom use, or when they suggest that Abstinence Plus sex education leaves out all aspects of feelings, is strictly mechanistic, and leaves parents out entirely.

Some have even said that Comprehensive Sexuality Education/Abstinence Plus encourages sex, and that students in A+ programs begin sexual intercourse earlier.[4]

None of these complaints is true. Quite the contrary. Successful comprehensive sexuality education courses include parents, quite rightly recognizing that they have an enormous influence over their children.

Successful courses emphasize communication and discussions about feelings; they teach teens how to say no just as they teach them how to use contraception safely. They encourage abstinence as the first and best choice. From the research point of view, the statistics on perfect condom use show a failure rate of 3 percent with perfect use, 14 percent with typical use.[5]

Factors in Choosing Abstinence

Why do some teens choose abstinence? Why do some choose to be sexually active? For teens, choosing abstinence or choosing to be sexually active is influenced by many factors. The influences, according to Advocates for Youth data:[6]

- The teen's age
- Physical maturity
- Aspirations
- Culture
- Participation in extracurricular activities
- School performance
- Religious beliefs
- Desire to avoid pregnancy and disease
- Family income
- Parental educational level
- Parental and personal values

"However," the report cautions, "adults should be aware that there is not a choice for every young person; for some, sexual intercourse is involuntary, a result of coercion, abuse, rape, or survival."[7] The statistics on sexual abuse, rape, incest, and male predators show that 74 percent of the women who had intercourse before age 14, and 60 percent of those who had sex before age 15 report having had sex involuntarily.[8]

Finally, all youth, whether abstinent or sexually active, deserve both accurate sexual health information and affordable contraceptive services.[9] Also important is a community that is teen-friendly, non-judgmental, and offers both counseling and access to services.

Other factors that influence the choice of abstinence are warmth, love and caring from parents or family; parental supervision; and two-parent homes.

Religion and prayer can also be important. According to teens who are involved in religious observance, their faith is an important reason for them to delay sex.

Dropouts from Abstinence Only Programs

A major problem with Abstinence Only programs concerns those teens who defect. Are they ostracized? Do they have access to information about contraception in the event they choose to have sex? Is someone there to advise and help them? And what about those who report themselves as abstinent but engage in oral sex, anal sex, or mutual masturbation? Are they practicing safer sex, even though it's not vaginal?

For *all* teens, we must have quality comprehensive sexuality education in place. An example of a successful comprehensive program is *Reducing the Risk: Building Skills to Prevent Teen Pregnancy, STDs, and HIV,* evaluated in California.[10] This high school course encompasses a broad program including sexuality education that stresses avoiding unprotected intercourse by abstinence or by using contraception. It encourages students to talk with their parents, accurately read risky situations, and visit stores and clinics.

The instructor uses role-play to teach decision making, negotiation, and responses to peer pressure. Research results indicate a delay in sexual activity as well as increased knowledge and contraceptive use among sexually active teens who have taken this course.

Postponing Sexual Involvement in Georgia and elsewhere[11] teaches decision making, negotiation skills, and responses to peer pressure, and is preceded by a human sexuality course including contraception. Evaluation shows participants are five times less likely to initiate sex by the end of the eighth grade than are those in the control group. Evaluation of a program that is modeled on PSI but does not include the sexuality unit showed no such changes.

Be Proud! Be Responsible! Strategies to Empower Youth to Reduce Their Risk for AIDS is a five-hour AIDS reduction intervention for 13-18-year-olds in the inner city. Behavioral findings indicate that after the intervention there is less risky sexual behavior, less sexual intercourse, and more consistent condom use.[12]

Adult training is essential, according to the Centers for Disease Control. They recommend sixteen hours for educators who are experienced in adolescent sexuality and HIV/AIDS, and 24 hours for those with less experience.

Working Through Our Differences

The chart on pages 116-117 shows many philosophical differences. Are we dreaming to think these two points of view can come to terms with each other for the benefit of our young people?

Perhaps we can't be entirely together philosophically. Perhaps we *can* come to a practical meeting of the minds and develop programs that will honor Abstinence Only while teaching it as part of the more inclusive Comprehensive Sexuality Education (Abstinence Plus).

Public support for sexuality education is at a high level, according to a poll commissioned by SIECUS (Sexuality Information and Education Council of the United States) and Advocates for Youth, Washington, DC.[13]

- Ninety-three percent of all Americans polled supported sexuality education in high schools.

- 84 percent showed such support in middle/junior high schools. Concern over teen pregnancy, HIV/AIDS, and other STIs appears to be the motivator.

- Of these Americans, *70 percent oppose the Abstinence Only government funded education* that prohibits the teaching of contraception.

- Eighty percent of the respondents do not believe that comprehensive sexuality education that includes the teaching of contraception encourages sexual activity.

- More than 90 percent support the teaching of abstinence as *part* of the comprehensive program.[14]

The poll confirmed that parents want the schools to be their partners in the sexuality education of their children and desire an Abstinence Plus approach.

The legislators are not hearing enough from the many people who support Abstinence Plus sexuality education that encourages the inclusion of abstinence skills as long as it does not deny students access to other contraceptive information. Parents must become involved at every level. Sexuality education must be

combined with parent-child communication, accessible teen-
friendly clinics, religious community involvement, committed
and caring youth-serving professionals, and effective media
messages. Parents and other caring adults need to speak up with
a loud clear voice.

Since risk reduction must be a piece of responsible sexuality
education as well as the skills of communication, negotiation,
and refusal, Abstinence Only cannot do the complete job. The
research confirms that comprehensive sexuality education
programs encourage abstinence, delay the initiation of intercourse, and increase the use of contraception. In other words,
it works.

Our goals should be clear: *delay sexual activity for safest
outcome; teach respect and responsibility for safer sex whenever
sexual activity begins.*

8

Sexuality Education — What's a School to Do?

I got into sex at 13 because I felt pushed out of the house when my mother had a baby. I found companionship with guys and decided it would be fun to try sex. If I'd had real sex education with feelings, discussions, explanations of contraception and how to get it, I wouldn't have gotten pregnant at 16.

Jessica, 17-year-old mother

Focus on Schools

In spite of strong public support for sexuality education in the schools, less than half of the states require the schools to provide it. About one-third provide Abstinence Only education with no contraceptive or disease prevention teaching. The majority voices favoring Comprehensive Sexuality Education (Abstinence Plus) are not being heard as clearly as the far fewer voices fighting for abstinence only.

"Most kids get some 'plumbing' sex ed on puberty, but less than ten percent of schools offer classwork on relationships, communication skills, feelings, contraception, sexual pleasure, sexual orientation, sexuality through the life cycle," commented Barbara Huberman, Advocates for Youth. Even rape, abuse, and sexual violence and victimization are frequently left out, she added.

The major argument about sexuality education revolves around school curricula, who teaches the courses, and the values taught. Religious leaders, youth leaders, politicians, parents, PTA/PTOs and school boards don't expect to do much about informal sex education. They don't get into what parents tell their children at home or what checkout clerks say to teens in drugstores, but they do get into classrooms and occasionally into school libraries.

To clarify my understanding of the values underlying the two kinds of education, I prepared the chart on the opposite page. It compares them on a variety of criteria.

In a democratic society we must honor diversity, tolerance, the spread of unrestricted information, and informed choice.

Social conservatives argue that comprehensive sexuality education that goes beyond teaching abstinence will lead to promiscuity and early sex while more moderate thinkers counter with statistics that refute this concept.[1] The World Health Organization (WHO) reviewed 35 sexuality programs. They found that Abstinence Only programs were less effective than programs that promoted the delay of first intercourse and also taught safer sex practices such as contraception and condom use. None increased the level of sexual activity. Some comprehensive programs showed decreases in activity and the number of partners plus a more effective use of contraception.[2] As mentioned before, data from the Netherlands where liberal sexuality education is built into the whole society, show that teens initiate sexual intercourse at a median age about one and a half years *later* than ours do, i.e. at almost age 18 compared with our median age of 16.3.[3]

Comparing Sexuality Education Programs		
	Abstinence Only (Abstinence Until Marriage)	**Comprehensive Including Abstinence (Abstinence Plus)**
Motivating force	Morality, politics	Health, safety
Sexual orientation stance	Homophobic	Accepting
Bias	Against teen sex	Against unprotected sex
Attitude	Judgmental	Neutral, supportive
Data	Inaccurate, worst-case	Research based
Method	Instill fear, obedience	Instill respect, responsibility
Information	Restricted	Generated, spread
Time line	Junior high, high school	K-12 preferred
Scope	Abstinence only	Abstinence-based, comprehensive, and whole person
Whose comfort level?	Adults	Children of all ages
Risk factor	High	Low
Philosophical base	Preset standard of behavior	Informed choice
Religious base	Conservative, traditional	Universal values
Goal	Delay sexual intercourse until high school graduation or until marriage	Delay sexual intercourse. Lower rates of teen pregnancy. Lower rates of STIs. Lower rates of abortion.
Evaluation	No case-controlled longitudinal studies show effectiveness	Case-controlled longitudinal studies show effectiveness

In spite of the political infighting, however, formal school-based sexuality education, taught with a planned curriculum, has been ongoing for years in America. There are very different emphases and access in various parts of the country depending on the socio-political attitudes of the people making the

decisions. Yet few programs are modeled after the European
approach that centers on what the students want to know.

Comprehensiveness Often Lacking

Sexuality education finds its way into schools in a variety of
formats. A life management skills course given in Florida high
schools includes some sexuality education.[4] Embedded in the
course are performance standards that cover topics such as teen
suicide, depression, cancer, wellness, the menstrual cycle,
hormones, methods of contraception, drug abuse, drug prevention, physical and emotional abuse, stress, career planning and
budgeting. The curriculum describes HIV/AIDS and other STIs,
and reviews their effects on the human body systems.

It describes and identifies ways of avoiding pregnancy and
STIs, but students are not asked to identify *actions* they can take
to avoid them. A standard on suicide says, "Identify *actions* an
individual can take to intervene in a potential and impending
suicide." A standard on pregnancy and STIs says, "Identify *the
methods* of avoiding (them) using current research, understanding that abstinence is the expected standard for school age
children."

Excellent as this course is in a number of areas, it doesn't
address the importance of prevention of conception and infection
by methods other than abstinence, even in high school programs
provided for pregnant and parenting teens. We are closing our
eyes to what is happening in the real world once again. We are
concentrating on what is perceived as "good curriculum," one
that fits our notion of what we think should, or should not, be
happening.

When we deal with "shoulds" and "oughts" we are not
dealing with reality. The negative outcome of this is that teens,
sensing a lecture coming, turn off and don't hear important
information they need.

Teens need to know how to prevent HIV/AIDS and unplanned
children as much if not more than they need to know how to
prevent health hazards from "additives, improper (food) storage
and preparation." The Florida life management course includes a

variety of learning styles, is obviously well thought out, and may be effective in teaching the skills needed for living a healthy life, *except for openness in the area of sexuality*. Here it skirts the real issues, the ones that could affect teens' lives the most. Most of the teens I interviewed told me that the only sexuality education that ever influenced them explored feelings and taught communication skills.

As important as knowledge is, true comprehensive education must also address attitudes, feelings, and skills. Students need to be free to question and explore their sexual stirrings. A teacher in Germany talked about this. She told us, "Whatever questions the students have are answered. We're not afraid of any topic." The high school students in the European countries we studied were also given careful instructions in the use of a condom. Just as important, they were taught the communication skills they would need to negotiate condom use with a partner.

Components of Successful Program

What are the programs that work the best? So far, we know that they are the comprehensive programs that include not only factual information, but open discussion about topics with which teens need help — how to:

- Say no.
- Negotiate the use of contraception and condoms.
- Find access to services.
- Remain abstinent with a support system of like-minded teens.
- Find mentors who will offer support through their adolescent years.
- Feel good about themselves as they increase their decision making skills.

Surely sexuality education must include the types, instruction for use, advantages and disadvantages of various kinds of contraception. It must teach teens how to access services and devices, including emergency contraception. Honest, open discussion of conception, contraception (starting with absti-nence), negotiation skills, and social skills offer the most effective means of protecting teens from infection, unplanned pregnancies, and abortion.

Tom Klaus, sexuality educator and consultant in Iowa, makes the point that it's important for teens to talk about sex with their prospective partners. They may be going into it for the purpose of pleasing the other, when neither may want it. The myth is that everyone is doing it; the reality is that not everyone wants to. Talking may be the best prevention.

Peer sexuality education is growing in importance as research confirms that teens are more likely to hear (and change) attitudes and behaviors if they believe the messenger is similar to them.[5] Peer programs that have been evaluated show that after structured programs by trained teens the following changes occurred:[6]

- An increased knowledge of HIV prevention.
- Increased condom use by sexually active teens who perceived that their peers use condoms.
- Lower rates of tenth graders initiating sex compared with the control groups.

Finding Effective Resources

Some of the most effective resources come from places other than curriculum planners in the schools. Robie H. Harris has written a sexuality education book, *It's Perfectly Normal,*[7] that would be an asset in every classroom from the fourth grade up. It would also be useful for adults all over our country. Each of us would find something to learn and to share with our children. It's an excellent example of the content of a good sexuality education course. It's honest, it puts up a mirror to ourselves, it's young person friendly, and it's clever and humorous. Both factual and serious, it builds on children's learning ability as it moves from the simple to the more complex. Above all, it's reassuring.

Another fine resource for districts seeking to implement a sexuality education program is Peggy Brick's *The New Teaching Safer Sex.*[8] She explains her rationale for the manual: "All the lessons . . . are designed to involve participants in active dialogue about sex. When taught in a supportive, non-judgmental environment, we find the strategies increase participants' comfort in talking about sexual issues as well as their knowledge and skills for practicing safe behaviors. Our goal is to create a climate where communication about sexuality is normal and the use of safer sex is the expected behavior."

Objectives include:

• Understanding the option *not* to engage in sexual behavior is a basic human right.

• Understanding the possible consequences of sexual intimacy, particularly when vaginal, oral or anal intercourse are involved.

• Knowing the actions that can be taken to reduce the risk of unwanted consequences.

• Developing knowledge, skill and comfort needed to practice safer sex.

• Assessing the risk involved in one's own sexual behavior.

• Setting goals to make safer sex an integral part of one's sex life.

• Developing the skills necessary to work cooperatively with a partner to assume responsibility for safer sex.

Brick comments, "When compared to young people in Western Europe who receive open, honest education and support for 'respectful and responsible' sexual behavior, our youth are disadvantaged."

Girls Incorporated Preventing Adolescent Pregnancy has four components: "Taking Care of Business," "Growing Together," "Will Power/Won't Power," and "Health Bridge." These programs combine caring mentors, an environment in which girls feel they belong together, and good education, all working to help teens make responsible decisions. Each addresses the information, skills and self-esteem females need to avoid early pregnancy. Together they cover career goals, parent/daughter communication, refusal skills, and health. A four-year evaluation found that participants in the whole curriculum were less likely to initiate early sexual intercourse.[9]

Our Whole Lives[10] is a series of sexuality education curricula for five age groups: K-1, grades 4-6, 7-9, 10-12, and adults. *Our Whole Lives* is designed to help participants make informed and responsible decisions about their sexual health and behavior. It provides accurate, age-appropriate information in human development, relationships, personal skills, sexual behavior, sexual health, and society and culture. The curricula provides facts about anatomy and human development. It also helps participants clarify their values, build interpersonal skills, and understand the spiritual, emotional, and social aspects of sexuality.

Our Whole Lives is appropriate for use in a variety of school and community settings, including classrooms, after-school programs, and youth groups. Although developed by the Unitarian Universalist Association and the United Church of Christ, the curricula contains no religious references or doctrine. An optional religious component is available, however, for faith-based settings.

The National Education Association Health Information Network also has jumped into the fray by producing a video and guide called "Considering Your Options,"[11] an educational video about contraceptive alternatives. Designed for high school use as part of a comprehensive health education program, it is teen friendly and should hold teens' attention. It faces the reality that by age 19 the majority of teens are sexually active, and it acknowledges that contraceptive information is essential for high school students. Its purpose is to provide teens with enough clear information to make informed decisions.

HIV/AIDS Curricula That Works

There are other evaluated curricula that work. The Centers for Disease Control has evaluated curricula in sexuality education and HIV/AIDS prevention. The following units have proven successful on a number of criteria.[12]

Get Real About AIDS (GRAA) is a fourteen-lesson school-based high school curriculum that is accompanied by a parents' newsletter. A key component is training. The developer of the program recommends three days of teacher training and four days of trainer training. This is a big commitment for a school district, but the results appear to be worth the time. The developer, The Comprehensive Health Education Foundation, will help schools arrange for training.

Twenty-three hundred students involved in the intervention conducted in Colorado scored significantly higher than the control group on a post-test of HIV knowledge. Other findings included sexually active students' intentions to practice safer sex, to have sex less often, and to use a condom when having intercourse. Intervention students, whether sexually active or not, were more likely to believe that their age group could become infected with HIV.

Becoming a Responsible Teen (BART) is an intervention that was conducted in a comprehensive community health center serving predominately low-income, minority residents in a southern urban area. Participants attended eight weekly sessions of a sexually explicit education program that included behavior skills, HIV/AIDS infection, correct condom use, assertive communication, refusal skills, information, self-management, problem-solving, and risk recognition. Groups were made up of five to fifteen adolescents separated by gender.

The findings were rewarding. Of the sexually abstinent youth involved in BART, only 11.5 percent were sexually active one year later compared with 31 percent of the adolescents in the control group. Of those sexually active prior to BART, only 27 percent in the intervention group remained so compared with 42 percent of the control group. BART participants were more likely to use condoms and less likely to engage in unprotected vaginal or anal intercourse. The BART group scored higher on the AIDS knowledge test and maintained that lead a year later. They were even more skillful in providing information to peers.

Informal Teaching

Formal curriculum in the schools is not enough. We need to enlarge our vision and add good sexuality education in creative ways. Every good teacher and parent knows there is a "teachable moment," a time in the classroom or family life when, if he or she seizes it, some real learning will take place. A cartoon shows children crowded around the gerbil cage watching baby gerbils being born. The science teacher calls them away saying, "Back to your seats, children, it's time for science!" Sexuality education can be very effective when it is integrated into other subjects in the curriculum.

Before they even get to the classroom, teens may find an example of sex education in a school library. A middle school in Hauppague, NY, removed three magazines aimed at teens — *YM, Teen,* and *Seventeen* — from the library shelves, citing their sexually oriented content as being inappropriate for students.[13] The student who discovers that these magazines have been banned finds a message on the empty shelf. Sex is bad. We can't expose young people to it. We have to protect them from information about it.

The magazines banned in this school library would have made wonderful curricula. Students, with the guidance of a mature teacher, could review them and talk about their content, evaluate the power of their messages to teens, and discuss the appropriateness of their being in the school library. These topics would engender real sexuality education, including decision-making, responsibility, respect, and relationships.

Respect Sexual Orientation

Sensitivity to the needs of gay, lesbian, bisexual and transgender youth is an essential part of comprehensive sexuality education. Because of the homophobia so prevalent in our society, these young people are at higher risk for HIV/AIDS and other STIs. The majority of adult lesbian and bisexual women have had heterosexual intercourse at some point in their lives, and at least 30 percent have been pregnant.[14]

According to a report from the Minnesota Adolescent Health Survey, bisexual and lesbian respondents were about as likely as heterosexual women ever to have had intercourse, but they had a significantly higher prevalence of pregnancy. Researchers suggest several possible reasons. Sexual abuse, incest, and rape are more prevalent among lesbian and bisexual young women than among heterosexual youth. Another possible reason is that young women who think they might be lesbian, and have accepted society's negative homophobic stereotype, have heterosexual intercourse to "prove" they are straight. Whatever the reason, providers of reproductive health care and family planning services should not assume that pregnant teens are heterosexual. They need to realize that gay, lesbian, bisexual, and transgender youth may also be in need of family planning and STI prevention services.

In fact, the Minnesota study results suggest that adolescent women who identify themselves as lesbian or bisexual, or unsure of their sexual orientation, may be at *increased* risk of pregnancy, repeat pregnancies, adverse pregnancy outcomes, and poor contraceptive practices.

About ten percent of any group of young people will eventually identify themselves as gay, lesbian, bisexual, or transgender. Schools, clinics, youth organizations, church groups, all who serve/work with/care about young people have an obligation to support and provide a safe environment for all, regardless of their sexual orientation. Respect for one another is crucial, regardless of differences.

Primary Education Concerning Sexuality

Over the last few years, some New Jersey school boards, and a few in other states, adopted a comprehensive early family life education model. It was created with the help of child development experts and published by the Rutgers University Press. *Learning About Family Life*[15] is a family life/sexuality education program tailored for kindergarten to third grade. This is a nontraditional approach, since typically sexuality education takes place in high school, less frequently in middle school. As our cultural environment has undergone radical changes in the past fifty years, educators have begun to focus on younger ages.

Ann Schurmann, MPH, program manager of the Network for Family Life Education, wrote *Baby Steps: Implementing Family Life Education in the Early Grades*[16] to describe the program and the barriers some boards encountered before using it. She cited some reasons board members used for adopting the program:

- The average age of menarche has declined with some girls beginning puberty as young as nine years old. It is important for children to learn about changes that take place at puberty before they happen.

- Children's culture, once surrounded only by comics and radio, now is inundated with sexual images and messages "many of which suggest that the more casual, reckless, and even exploitative sex is the more pleasurable."

- With sexual abuse rampant in our society, children must be openly educated about sex in order to better protect themselves.

- Teens, who are becoming sexually active at younger and younger ages, need protection from STIs and unintended pregnancy.

With a strong base in early childhood education, with a knowledge of child sexual development, with a fine, sensitive touch, and despite significant controversy in four of the twenty districts in which it was to be taught, the project was implemented. Topics covered are interpersonal relationships, human development, sexuality and reproduction, responsible personal behavior, and building strong families. It's a great resource for other school districts who agree that implementing family life education in the earliest grades is a good thing.

Barriers to implementation included the environment of a district, community controversy, fear of negative parental response, and teacher discomfort. Advocates for this project were able to overcome all of these, using a combination of patience, tact, and parental and teacher education.

Since implementation can be difficult, Schurmann recommends:

1. Go slowly.
2. Don't be overly cautious.
3. Have a plan.

4. Be open.
5. Obtain the support of your administration.
6. Educate adults first — teachers, parents, administrators.
7. Don't assign classroom teachers to teach this topic unless you can afford to provide them with adequate training.
8. If you're challenged, don't back down.

The keys seem to be openness, providing information and education, enlisting support you can count on, and being patient. Or, as we used to say in the teachers' room, do your homework.

Teaching the Teachers

The best program is only as good as the teacher who presents it. There are many excellent teachers. They are comfortable with their own sexuality and sensitive to students' developmental issues. Ideas and feelings are explored, skills are taught, and students feel secure. They see sexuality education as a part of their schooling whether it is taught as a separate subject or embedded in other subjects.

But not all teachers are comfortable. Some are not even willing, but are recruited because there is no one else to do it. When "Sex Ed" was introduced into my school system in the early 70s, fifth grade was selected as the best place to begin. Fifth grade teachers were pressed into service. Training began with an exploration of all the "words" in the curriculum that would be needed to communicate with the students. The low buzz in the room reached a crescendo as teachers realized they were expected to say — out loud — words that they had only whispered up to that time. That's when the real training began.

A SIECUS study, *Teaching Our Teachers to Teach,*[17] revealed that few teachers receive the training they need to be qualified as sexuality educators. Colleges and universities are not adequately preparing their students in HIV/AIDS prevention and comprehensive sexuality education.

There are places in our country where difficulties have been overcome. There are places where open and honest sexuality education is in place. There are places where the statistics have come way down through a combination of good sexuality education including both abstinence and information about contraception as well as accessibility to these services. And there are people who have come to realize the importance of protecting our children.

But there are places where the teen pregnancy and STI statistics remain high, show no sign of dropping, and where sexuality education is either prohibited or ignored. It is not enough for us to have *some* places where sexuality education is working. All of our children, and our adults, need to be reached so that we can, countrywide, lower the rates of teen pregnancy, of abortion, of STIs, and of unplanned births to teens. In this way, we can develop a society of sexually healthy people *who take responsibility for their own and their partner's health and well-being.*

CHAPTER

9

Contraception — "It Just Happened"

"It just happened."

I asked teen after teen, from 13-year-olds to 17-year-olds, "How did you happen to get pregnant?"

"It just happened."
"We didn't plan it."
"I never thought it could happen to me."
"I didn't think about it."
"We forgot."

"What did you know about contraception?" I asked.
"I didn't know about it."
"We couldn't get any."
"He didn't want to use it."
"The condom broke."

One young mother, then 15, told me that after she had her baby at 14 her mother took her to a doctor to get the pill. If she had known about it before she had sex, she said, she wouldn't have gotten pregnant.

"Did you know that, in addition to getting pregnant, you could also get a sexually transmitted infection, including HIV that causes AIDS?"

They seemed to understand this a little better, but again, *"Yeah, I heard about it, but I knew it couldn't happen to me."*

The above dialog would not have occurred in the Netherlands, France, or Germany.

As Berne and Huberman point out,[1] "In all three nations, adults encourage teens to be responsible about sex. National healthcare in each country covers the costs of most forms of contraception, emergency contraception, abortion, counseling services, physical exams, screening, and treatments. Condoms are inexpensive and widely available.

"All levels of healthcare personnel, including those staffing front desks, work hard to reduce or remove barriers that deter young people from getting needed health services and to establish and maintain a high degree of trust between young people and health practitioners. Educators, media professionals, and communities collaborate to motivate young people to recognize the benefits of responsible sexual behavior and to acquire and use contraception."

U.S. Adults Are Failing Teens

Shall we blame our young people for not being responsible? No, it's time we talk about *adult* failure rather than condom failure or teen failure. Teens I spoke with didn't know enough about contraception:

• The methods, how each functions and its effectiveness.

• Where to get contraception and what it costs.

• How to use them.

• How to negotiate with a partner about contraception.

• The responsibility everyone who engages in sex has to oneself, to a partner, and to the family they might be starting.

The teens didn't know enough about respect and the relationship between passion and love, between drive and commitment, between freedom and responsibility. And why not? Because we haven't taught them.

There are many examples of adult failure:

- Education that exposes them to the paternalistic, unrealistic notion that if they don't know anything, they'll be protected.

- Parents who either can't or don't choose to talk with their young children about sexuality.

- Schools that either shy away from sex education or give in to political pressure to water it down.

- Religious institutions that push the traditional Abstinence Only approach or choose to ignore the issues of teen sexuality altogether.

- Entertainment that pummels them with sexual fantasy.

Even though we have not been addressing positive and responsible teen sexuality vigorously enough, our society has changed. Women are no longer sheltered by chaperones, protected by strong marriage conventions, and restrained by societal attitudes that conferred shame on unwed motherhood. Since the advent of the pill, legalized abortion, the sexual revolution, and the women's movement, standards have changed for women of all ages. In fact, the standards of young women today were established by the older women they emulate. Consider the sexual role modeling of Hollywood and rock music, sex without consequences.

Contraceptives — Myths and Facts

A conference, "Messengers and Methods for the New Millennium: a Round Table on Adolescence and Contraception," was held in Washington, DC, in February, 1999. People there *were* thinking about the consequences. Among the presenters was Robert A. Hatcher, MD, MPH, professor of gynecology and obstetrics, Emery University School of Medicine. Dr. Hatcher spoke about a book he and his colleagues had developed for medical personnel who deal with contraception. He left each of us his gift, *A Pocket Guide to Managing Contraception.*[2] And what a gift it is!

This fit-in-the-pocket book was adapted from a large medical resource book available to professionals. Dr. Hatcher and his colleagues found the resource book too cumbersome and too inaccessible to providers in the field. Their goal was to make *A Pocket Guide* truly useful. It is written for healthcare providers, but it is equally helpful for teachers, social workers, teen sexuality educators, and parents who lead teens into a discussion of contraception.

Chapter One introduces "Adolescent Issues." Teens are often uncomfortable discussing sexual issues, he tells us. He suggests asking the question, "What are you doing to protect yourself from AIDS?" to prompt a healthy dialogue about sexuality and to guide advice on contraception. Dr. Hatcher dispels misconceptions many young people have:

- You can't get pregnant the first time you have intercourse.
- You can't get pregnant without penetration.
- If you have not yet had a period, you can't get pregnant.
- You can't get pregnant if you douche after sex.

The truths are:
- You can get pregnant the first time.
- Seminal fluid outside the vagina can enter it and cause pregnancy.
- Ovulation can occur before the onset of menses.
- Douching does not kill all semen.

What eye openers for teens who have heard the myths but don't know the truths. And what a wonderful way to begin instruction on contraception! He further points out that nearly all teens are legally entitled to confidential services and counseling. Given the amount of highly charged political infighting over this issue, many teens aren't aware of this fact.

Communication between partners about the use of contraception is vital. Girls don't get pregnant by themselves.

Just as they need a male partner to get pregnant, so do they need a male partner to help prevent pregnancy. Men tend to be older than their partners, and older males are less likely to use contraception at first sex.[3]

Assuming that such sex is voluntary, young women need to learn how to negotiate the use of contraception. Males need help, too, preferably from adult men, role models in comfortable and familiar settings.

Menu of Contraceptives

An honest presentation of the risks and the ways to prevent the risks is far better than resorting to scare tactics. In the chapter, "Choosing Between Available Contraceptives,"[4] Dr. Hatcher stresses the multidimensionality of contraception. He describes variations, advantages and disadvantages in each of the methods:

- abstinence
- withdrawal
- calendar
- the pill
- IUD
- male condoms
- female condoms
- spermicide
- diaphragm
- Depo-Provera
- Norplant
- sterilization
- emergency contraceptive pills.

He notes that in making choices, people should be aware of their own biases. He points out that convenience and the ability to use the method correctly are important, and that people must be able to negotiate with a partner over the need for contraception. All good material for teen providers.

Teen failure to use condoms correctly results in part from the lack of sexuality education on correct and consistent use. Yet the opposition insists, "Teach them how to use them? Why not teach them how to have sexual intercourse right in class? That's what you're encouraging."

As mentioned before, we have clear and consistent data showing us that in those countries that include this kind of contraceptive education in their sexuality education classes, the median age for initiation of sex is between one and two years *later* than our median age.

In this country studies have shown that among teens who have comprehensive sexuality education, the numbers of sexually active teens do *not* rise. We also know that when teens do engage in sex, they are far more likely to protect themselves if they know how to do so.

It is clear that abstinence is the only 100 percent sure method of pregnancy and STI prevention. The pill comes close with a nearly 100 percent success rate when used perfectly, a 95 percent success rate with a typical user.[5] It still does nothing to prevent infection. Condoms also *must* be used if either partner is not STI free, has not been tested and found clear of HIV, and/or there is the slightest chance their relationship is not monogamous.

Abstinence is the clear winner in pregnancy and disease prevention. Too often, however, the abstinence-only message includes teaching that contraceptives, especially condoms, have a high failure rate. This is not true. As reported earlier, the male condom correctly and perfectly used has a 3 percent failure rate. It is when condoms are used inconsistently, or used incorrectly that there is a higher failure rate.[6]

When most people think of contraception, they think of the male condom and the pill. However, Depo-Provera, given by injection, is becoming more well known and more widely used.[7] Depo-Provera, a contraceptive injection introduced into the market in 1995, now accounts for 19 percent of contraceptive use among African American teens, slightly less than 19 percent use among Hispanic teens, and 8 percent among non-Hispanic white teens. Its acceptability to teens, especially those from lower income families, is credited to the simplicity of use and its nearly 100 percent effectiveness.

Depo-Provera is considered an important contributor to the

marked decline in teen pregnancies, especially among unmarried African American women.[8]

More people may begin to use this contraceptive as they recognize its efficacy.

Many teens choose the privacy of Depo-Provera because they fear abuse from partners; others don't want to disappoint parents. And the big reason — they don't have to think about it every day as they do with the pill — although they *must* get the injection every 90 days.[9]

Norplant, tiny capsules inserted surgically into the upper arm, is highly effective for those who want an even longer period of preventive coverage. Its success rate was documented at one pregnancy per 20,000 perfect use users in the first year.[10] Norplant is expensive, but offers protection from pregnancy for five years. With Norplant, however, it is important that the user has a competent healthcare provider who can remove the implants when she desires.

Although not every type of contraception appeals to every young person who chooses to become sexually active, it is important that they know their options and understand the advantages and disadvantages of each. In addition, it must be stressed that although each of these prevents pregnancy, only the condom prevents STIs.

The Dutch have popularized the "Double Dutch" method, the pill or other contraceptive for birth control, and the condom for infection control. In the United States the research tells us that as males realize the female is using the pill, they tend to discontinue use of the condom. This is pre-STI thinking when many people were concerned only with pregnancy. Now it is imperative that both partners be concerned with infections, particularly HIV, both for themselves and the children they may produce.

Emergency Contraception

Emergency contraception pills (ECPs), are little known, underused, and widely misunderstood. The Food and Drug Administration has approved their marketing and sale,[11] and researchers have known about them for more than twenty years.

Yet few American doctors have offered guidance on them. Most people don't know about them, and if they do, they don't know how to get them.

Emergency contraception is a woman's last chance to prevent or delay ovulation after unprotected sex. Most commonly, it involves taking higher than usual numbers of birth control pills within 72 hours of unprotected intercourse, followed by another dose twelve hours later.[12]

The press and anti-abortion advocates have publicized ECPs as "abortion." Research has shown, however, that although they are 75 percent effective in preventing *ovulation* if used within 72 hours after unprotected sex, they will *not* terminate an established pregnancy.

The lack of understanding about this method is unfortunate. Abortion foes can take comfort from the fact that consistent use of this method (in cases of slippage or breakage of condoms or of involuntary sex) could prevent 800,000 abortions per year.[13] Now approved in the United States, drug manufacturers are packaging ECPs specifically for use as emergency contraception.

We need education around the issue of emergency contraception as much as we need it around traditional contraception. A 1997 survey[14] reported that 66 percent of women and 51 percent of men knew about ECPs, but only one percent used them, and only eleven percent knew what to do with them. Part of the education, according to professionals, should be that they not be seen as a regular method of contraception since they are not as effective, are more expensive, and have side effects such as nausea and vomiting.

Nor should they, like any other birth control pill, be seen as effective against HIV/AIDS or other sexually transmitted infections. The most effective protection is a condom plus a female contraceptive, plus an ECP in the event of an accident.

The American Medical Women's Association[15] is advocating for ECPs to be available over the counter. They see them as safe, effective, and far more accessible if sold in drugstores without a prescription.

Contraception Is Effective

What are the facts on adolescent contraceptive use? According to the Advocates for Youth publication, *The Facts,* November, 1998:[16]

- Each year 1.7 million adolescent pregnancies are averted by the use of contraceptives, 1.5 million of these by oral contraceptives alone. These prevented pregnancies could have resulted in about 737,000 abortions. Both pro-life and pro-choice advocates can cheer these results.

- Adolescents who have received contraceptive education are 33 percent more likely to use some form of contraception than those who have not. It makes sense, of course, that if you are about to engage in sexual intercourse and you know how to protect yourself, you are more likely to do that. If you are about to have sexual relations and you have no idea how to protect yourself, or if you have been taught it is wrong to use contraceptives, you are not likely to protect yourself.

- Emergency contraception can prevent 74 to 80 percent of unintended pregnancies from unprotected intercourse.

- Adolescent women whose partners are within two years of their own age are more likely to use contraception (80.9 percent) than teens whose first partner is five or more years older (66 percent). Common sense would suggest that older men would be even more aware of the need for contraception, and have the means of obtaining it, than would younger males. Though they put their partners at far greater risk of contracting STIs because of their own longer period of sexual relationships, older men are less likely than teenagers to use condoms. If for no other reason than this, young women should be wary of sexual relations with older men.

- Communication is a significant factor in safer sex. Students who discuss HIV with their parents are less likely to have unprotected sex or multiple partners.

- Positive parental and peer role models of healthy behavior also contribute to greater use of contraceptives among teens.

Is there good news on the teen pregnancy front? Child Trends indicates that teen pregnancy rates have dropped to their lowest rate in two decades, down from 117 pregnancies per 1,000 teens in 1990 to 97 per 1,000 teens in 1996.[17]

The Centers for Disease Control attribute the recent decline in teen birth and pregnancy rates to a leveling off of sexual experience and activity and to increased condom use among sexually active youth. Experts attribute 80 percent of the decline to improved use of highly effective, long acting contraceptives by sexually active teenagers, accompanied by increased condom use. They attribute 20 percent of the decline in the overall teen pregnancy rate to increased abstinence.[18]

How are we doing? If there is greater use of contraceptives and fewer teens are having sex, we're doing better than we were, and that's the good news. But the lack of contraceptive coverage in health insurance makes some effective forms of contraception too expensive for many women. This leads to unintended pregnancies.[19] Several public programs fund these services, including federal services such as Medicaid, Title X, maternal and child health block grants, and social service block grants, with state funds making up the difference.

Are these services effective? They prevent between 1.2 million and 2.1 million unplanned pregnancies a year.[20]

Yet, so shortsighted are we that total public expenditures for contraceptive services decreased steadily from 1980 to 1992 before rising again. Title X of the Public Health Service Act, the Federal Family Planning Program, serves large numbers of teens with reproductive health issues, but is controversial because of public attitudes toward adolescent pregnancy. Although proponents argue for expansion to help reduce the rate of unintended pregnancies, critics question its effectiveness.

Title X continues to be funded, but amendments continue to be proposed that include parental notification and consent. Since we know that teens shun services where they fear their confidentiality will be breached, such passage could defeat the teen pregnancy prevention purpose of Title X.[21] The Alan Guttmacher Institute reports that every public dollar spent for family planning services saves an average of $3 in Medicaid costs for pregnancy-related health care.[22] Perhaps this will convince legislators of the efficacy of Title X.

We're making some progress with federal law. Under a new statute, the Federal Employees' Health Benefits Program is required to include coverage of prescription contraceptives under their prescription drug coverage.[23] There had been a skirmish about including it, but the proponents won out. This sets a good example for other health insurers.

Making Contraception Legitimate

According to Dr. Laurie Schwab Zabin, professor at Johns Hopkins School of Hygiene and Public Health, the single most important issue concerning contraception is its perceived legitimacy of use. She reports that since over 90 percent of United States women say they use contraception, we think of ourselves as a contraceptive society. "But," she questions, "are we? Our figures on unintended pregnancy belie our claim." She believes that the increase in condom *awareness* is due to fear of HIV, and she reports that males are now using condoms in large numbers.

The real question for the United States, according to Dr. Zabin, is why contraceptive use is less efficient, less acceptable, and less successful here than it is in the rest of the developed world. She attributes this to "two critical underlying reasons":

• Children are undervalued in our society.
• Contraception is distrusted and undervalued in terms of its safety and efficacy.

Everything we do in terms of policy, service, delivery, and the messages in the public discourse serve to take away from instead of adding to contraception's legitimacy. She points out that singling out adolescents is not an appropriate strategy.

Dr. Zabin reports, "Eighty percent of our school-based clinics don't offer contraception. Campaigns waste pregnancy prevention dollars to tell teens they don't want to be pregnant, which teens already tell us. Abstinence teaching often implies that having sex leads to pregnancy without mentioning any responsible intervening choice. All these strategies delegitimize contraception. These are not benign missed opportunities; they countermand the message we should be sending. If parents are dubious about use, how can they convince teens? If partners can't talk with each other about it, how can they use it?"

She calls for a national campaign that addresses the two critical dimensions of reproductive responsibility:

• The importance of children and childbearing.
• The safety and efficacy of contraception.

"Both messages must be directed at *all* ages, not only at teens, as this would be so much more acceptable. We don't direct the seat belt message to children alone, we direct it to everyone. We need to make the use of contraception and the avoidance of having a child as an accident so much a part of the culture that young people hear it growing up. Until we can talk about it publicly and strongly, we certainly can't convince them," she said.

Dr. Zabin ended with a quote from a clergyman, "Fornication is a sin, but bringing an unwanted life into the world is a greater sin."

If we truly respect life, *our unwillingness to wholeheartedly prevent the getting or giving of sexually transmitted infections and the begetting of unwanted children is immorality at its highest level.*

10

HIV, AIDS, STIs —
Alphabet of Pain

The scene: The Orderly Room at the Army base in San Luis Obispo, California, as the eighteen-year-old soldiers are getting ready to go on leave for the night. A large bowl of condoms on the First Sergeant's desk, the gruff voiced Sergeant standing over it. "Boys, you don't leave this room without a condom!"

Most of the boys shrugged their shoulders, raised their eyebrows, and stuffed the condom into the back pocket of their uniform pants. But one boy stood fast, shaking his head. "I can't. I can't," he said over and over.

"Why in Hell not?" roared the First Sergeant.

"Because I'm Catholic, and I can't take a condom."

"Then you're not going on leave," said the Sergeant.

His friends talked with him, encouraging him to take one so he could go out with them. "Take it and throw it away. Don't use it. He won't know," they said to him.

"Come on, it's getting late. Let's go."
But the soldier stood firm, turned around and went back
into the barracks. The year — 1944.

When two World War II veterans told me this story, I asked them what they thought about the whole idea of being forced to take condoms. "If you had seen the movies they showed us with the syphilis and gonorrhea sores and other infections, you'd have thought it was a good idea to take one."

"Why do you suppose they were so strict about the whole thing?" I asked.

"They told us, 'We have to take care of you boys'."

Protection from Disease *More* Important Today

Over 50 years ago we were onto something about taking care of our young people, our boys in uniform, the boys who, though teens, were old enough to fight a war. And here we are, half a century later, with at least eight more identified STIs[1] (sexually transmitted infections, formerly called sexually transmitted diseases or STDs), with the worldwide scourge of HIV and AIDS. Rates of STIs for U.S. teens are four to twenty times higher than teens in other Western countries. We're not taking this challenge now as seriously as we did then. Aren't our young people as valuable to us now as they were when we needed them to fight a war?

Have our deep feelings of shame about these issues made us unwilling to acknowledge them? If we ignore them maybe they'll go away. But this silence has contributed to their persistence, even though we know we have the capability of decreasing or eliminating disease.[2] European countries, notably the Netherlands, France, and Germany, have significantly lowered their STI rates because of their pragmatic approach to sexuality. They have educated the public through schools and through mass media campaigns.

Why is it so important that we mobilize our whole society in our campaign to lower the rates of sexually transmitted diseases? There are many good reasons:[3, 4, 5]

- "Old" STIs are not gone and new ones have been identified since 1980.
- Knowledge about STIs is very low.
- High poverty level is a predictor of risk behavior.
- The age of puberty has fallen, making the years of risk even longer.
- Nearly 70 percent of our twelfth graders have engaged in sexual intercourse, half of it unprotected.
- Teens, particularly females, are highly susceptible to HIV and other sexually transmitted infections.
- Our STI rates are staggeringly high, higher than any other developed country.
- New risk behaviors involving needles such as tattooing and body piercing have become popular.
- Drug use with the sharing of needles and alcohol use with sex have not abated.
- The politics surrounding sex education and access to contraception has prohibited the kind of national campaign we need to bring about change.

Even those of us willing to talk about this topic do not have enough knowledge.[6] Some people think our only current problem is HIV and AIDS, but this is not true. We are still battling the diseases the government was worried about when they protected our servicemen in WWII, as well as the new STIs identified since that time.

Teens in the United States contract about 3 million STIs each year. Chlamydia is on the rise, with severe consequences. Our gonorrhea rate is 25 times higher than Germany. In the general population, the United States rate of AIDS is ten times higher than the rate in the Netherlands, thirteen times higher than Germany, and more than four times higher than the rate in France.[7] One in five people in the United States has an STI. About 25 percent of sexually experienced adolescents are infected.[8]

How many of these sexually transmitted infections can you name? If you can't list at least three, you have a lot of company. When the American Social Health Association asked 1,000 people in each of six countries if they could name one STI, an average of 33 percent could not. When the researchers then asked if they could name three or more STIs, Sweden scored highest with 48 percent. The United States was second with 23 percent. England, France, Italy, and Spain all had lower percentages, with Italy showing zero percentage of respondents naming three STIs.[9] Although most people knew about gonorrhea and syphilis, many had not heard of genital herpes, chlamydia, and genital warts.

Teens at Risk for STIs

Even if they don't know the names of these infections, over half of our teens may have been exposed to all of them by the time they become seniors in high school. Well, you might say, they're approaching adulthood by that time. Isn't it their problem? Yes it is, but public health is a problem for all of us, and the costs to society, especially to treat HIV/AIDS for a lifetime, are staggering. It becomes more of a problem as teens become sexually active earlier than they might have years ago.

This is partly because the age of menarche has decreased during the past century. Puberty, which used to occur on average between 13 and 15, now occurs between 10 and 13.[10] Sexually active young people engaging in unprotected sex are exposed to STIs at younger ages and for more years, increasing their risk each year.[11]

Yet another reason our young people are more at risk than those in the European countries mentioned above is the religious fundamentalist presence here in our politics, a movement that has grown over the past two decades. Many Abstinence Only advocates believe that educating young people about sex and about contraception will encourage them to have sex. Even adults who approve of making condoms available to teens often have mixed feelings. They fear they are giving a mixed message, "I don't want you to have sex, but here are some condoms because I know you will." Multiple studies disprove the concept that having condoms available *causes* teens to initiate sexual intercourse.[12]

In the United States, because of political pressure on law-makers and educators, we lack the following *national* research-based policies and systems that could delay sexual activity for some and provide protection for others:

• Fully comprehensive sex education K-12.

• Access to supportive family planning clinics that allow young people to get contraception and information without parental permission.

• A public media campaign that educates old and young alike to support "Safer Sex or No Sex."

• Non-judgmental attitude about teen sexuality.

• Public health policies based on scientific research, not politics or religious belief.

The American Social Health Association recommends that both partners, if they have had sex before, be tested for HIV and other STIs[13] before the initiation of intercourse, and that for each act of sexual intercourse they should use a new condom. They explode the myth that condom failure is the major cause of STI infection. It is unprotected sex or inconsistent or incorrect use of condoms.

The failure is not in the condom. It's a failure in trust. It's either adult failure to teach or teen failure or lack of opportunity to learn. What does it matter who's at fault when a young life has been so seriously, and often fatally, affected?

Teens, along with adults, are having a difficult time thinking about condoms and their use. A YWCA booklet announcing a teen prevention workshop includes quotes that help explain the condom phobia we have in this country.[14]

A young woman: "What I look like is more important than what I do. If I get taken advantage of it's my fault. If I enjoy sex I'm a nympho. If I am physically close with someone or am attractive but don't have sex I'm a mama's girl or a tease. If I have sex or carry condoms I'm a whore."

A young man: "If I chase girls I am a dog and a pig. If I like romance it must be because I just want to get a girl into bed. I am either religious, ugly, scared, a faggot, or a mama's boy if I just want to be close to a girl without having sex."

A *young woman:* *"I'm interested in having sex but how can I carry condoms or talk about sex when I know I'm not supposed to? I'll just let the other person worry about protection."*

A *young man:* *"I really don't like this person, we haven't gotten tested for HIV and don't have condoms, but I'm already 16 and I haven't had sex yet."*

What do these teens tell us about the norms of our society? The messages young people are getting from the sexuality education we do have, from the media, from parents, and from each other are so mixed and so confusing that they scarcely know what to do. If they want to remain virgins, they are scoffed at by some of their peers. If they want to have sex they don't know how to protect themselves.

Communication? Most teens just don't talk about sex, not to parents and certainly not to each other in a relationship. And condoms? They fear them, they suspect them, and they don't want to be tainted by them. They are, once again, reflecting adult attitudes toward condoms.

Normalizing Condom Use

The need to instill a new attitude into *all* sexually active Americans is never clearer than when we look at the research showing reasons teens don't use condoms with consistency:[15, 16]

- Negative peer perceptions about condoms.
- Decreased sexual pleasure.
- Unfamiliarity with use.
- No negotiation skills to use with a partner.
- Lack of availability.
- Cost factor.
- Lack of impulse control.
- Perceived invulnerability.
- The perception that condoms spoil the mood.
- Influence of alcohol and other drugs.

Of all the reasons given for teens not using condoms, peer attitude appears to be the most prevalent and the most influential. Teens don't think it's "cool." This is the area in which a heavy duty, consistent media campaign could make a big difference.

Look at how we sensitized our population to smoking. Once smoking was commonplace, but now a smoker in a restaurant might be glared at, even if he or she is in the smoking area. What used to be considered the norm is now frowned upon by non-smokers.

We did it with smoking, we did it with drunk driving, and we did it with seat belts. If we could make a difference in these areas that are less lethal overall than the spread of sexually transmitted infections, we can surely do it with condoms. Using a condom during intercourse needs to be the "in" thing to do.

Here's where the media campaign comes in. Everybody in the Netherlands, in France, and in Germany, when they are old enough to turn on the TV, knows about "Safer Sex or No Sex." The ads run with consistency, and they are well done. They are often aired free by the stations, more often publicly funded by the government.

They show condoms as part of any sexual encounter — it's respectful, it's responsible, it shows you care. Even more than that, if you don't use condoms, you are not "with it." Condoms are shown with all age groups and in normal, realistic situations.

They have taken it upon themselves to educate the public, and to make condom use "cool." A Dutch teen has it all figured out by the time he or she reaches puberty. It's as much a part of the culture as which sneakers are in style, or which jeans. They know they are expected to use condoms if they are sexually active, and they do.

Recently I listened to a teen forum in Washington, attended by French exchange students. They were amazed to see lots of TV ads against smoking, ads against drunk driving, ads promoting seat belt use, but no TV ads at all about "Safer Sex or No Sex."

"Where are the condom ads?" they asked. Where indeed.

Strategies for Helping Young People

Another area of concern has to do with young people who have found methods of having sex without "having sex." They maintain their virginity by not penetrating the vagina, but they expose themselves to possible infection in other ways. Oral sex, anal sex, and mutual masturbation have become ways to be close without having vaginal intercourse. The woman is still technically a virgin. But since both oral sex and anal sex can transmit STIs, the risk without protection is similar to vaginal sex. More education is needed in this area, too.

In education, what do we know about what doesn't work? We know that didactic teaching — "Just say 'No'" — is not nearly as effective as interactive strategies, i.e., identifying risky situations, skill in saying no, knowing how to use condoms, and learning how to negotiate their use with a partner. We also know from research that telling teens about the health risks of not using them, instilling fear about AIDS and other diseases, doesn't work.[17] Even though they appear to understand the message, and even though the adults themselves are moved by this argument, teens are convinced of their invulnerability. Their limited experience conditions them to believe that they are immortal. They don't think it can happen to them, no matter how risky their behavior.

What does work is a society's ability to influence youth through strategies such as multi-faceted media and public education campaigns. Prevention efforts should enlist the services of doctors and nurses as counselors and teachers, rather than only as medical care providers. School-based sex education needs to be comprehensive, K-12, and interactive. It should include abstinence as the safest contraception, with complete information on contraception and disease protection if not abstinent. Less formal education should come from peers, celebrities, sports stars, and others that teens want to emulate.

Adolescents who know how to get condoms, how to ask for them, how to use them, and how to negotiate with a partner about their use are far more likely to be consistent users. Perception of peer norms as supportive of condom use is the big one, and nothing works better than education given by caring and knowledgeable mentors, particularly those who are slightly older peers.

Teens who are especially inconsistent in condom use are those who don't believe that condoms will protect them from STIs. This belief may be the result of campaigns that claim condoms don't work. Respondents who understand that condom use *is* effective in preventing HIV transmission are 2.2 times more likely to be consistent in their use.[18]

Long-Term Benefits

We should not be surprised that impulsive teens respond to short-term benefits such as ease of use, rather than long term benefits such as staying healthy.[19] After all, unlike adults, they haven't had long lives in which to evaluate what long term benefits really can mean.

But adults *are* influenced by long-term benefits. In addition to the social benefits, we need to sell the economic benefits in lowering STI rates. In the United States, the estimated annual cost of major STIs is nearly $17 billion. These costs are more than 45 times greater than the dollars currently dedicated to prevention and 94 times greater than our investment in research in this area.[20] These staggering costs are attributable to the lack of prevention and to the fact that infections are not treated early enough.

Nearly three-fourths of the $1.5 billion cost of chalmydia is due to complications that could have been prevented if the infection had been diagnosed and treated earlier. Current federal funding for chlamydia reaches less than 20 percent of women at-risk in 30 states and 50 percent of at-risk women in the remaining states. Where funding and programs have been established, the program has reduced chlamydia rates by 66 percent and decreased treatment costs by 80 percent.[21]

We are back to our biggest problem with STIs, our reluctance to face the issue and address the problems. People say things to themselves like, "Not me. I'm fine," especially if they have no symptoms. So things get worse, harder to treat, and more expensive. Earlier diagnosis and treatment could save billions of dollars. Yet, like the U.S. policy with teen pregnancy, we don't put enough money or other resources into practical, realistic prevention initiatives.

Deadly Spread of AIDS

Homophobia and fear of public ridicule played a major role in our inaction and lack of urgency in reacting to the initial news about HIV and AIDS. When we first became aware of the disease in the early eighties, some who were heterosexual said, "Oh, it's the gay disease. No need to worry about me."

Others said, "It's their disease, and what did they expect?"

Still others commented, "It's their disease and it serves them right."

AIDS, now in its 18th year, is still spreading. It is pandemic in Africa and is making its way through large countries like India, China, and Brazil, where the huge populations result in a faster spread of disease.[22] Poverty, crowded conditions, lack of education, and lack of access to contraception all play a role. But of all of these, perhaps the ones most responsible for the spread are ignorance about who is really at risk, along with the homophobic attitudes that deny the problem or deny the solutions.

The data tell us otherwise. AIDS continues to spread. Estimates of AIDS cases in the United States by the Centers for Disease Control in 1998 are between 650,000 and 900,000. At least 40,000 new infections occur each year. Incidence is increasing most rapidly among heterosexuals. Women and African Americans are being infected disproportionately with the most dramatic increases in the South.[23]

These statistics exploded another myth about AIDS, that it's a city disease. No more. The most steady increase is taking place in rural areas.[24] Why so? Experts say it's people's lack of knowledge about risk and controversy over preventive measures such as clean-needle exchange programs and school-sponsored condom programs. Not too different from the controversy over teen pregnancy prevention.

Another big factor in the spread of AIDS in rural areas, according to Judy Glynn, AIDS activist, Axtel, Kansas, is the high social acceptance of drinking plus peer pressure to drink. "The drug of alcohol is more dangerous in our area and much more prevalent than shared needle use," she said. "Kids who wouldn't think of 'shooting up' don't hesitate to 'booze it up.'"

Still, there are gains being made in AIDS treatment. This should make us feel better, but it has created new problems.[25] The powerful new drugs, called cocktails, have lowered the death rate from AIDS in the United States by 29 percent in 1996 and 47 percent in 1997, the largest single year decline recorded for any major disease. Sounds wonderful except that:

- The drugs are prohibitively expensive.
- We still have 650,000 to 900,000 Americans with the HIV virus, and at least 40,000 new infections occur each year.
- As infected individuals live longer lives and have more energy, there is increasing danger that they will pass the virus on to others.
- As people hear of new "cures," they become complacent and return to unsafe sexual practices.

Challenge of Educating Teens About HIV/AIDS

At least half of new HIV cases are young people, with a disproportionate number of African Americans ages 15 to 44. In the United States, one of every four cases of AIDS was infected as a teenager. From a disease associated with gay whites, a group that is showing declining HIV rates, HIV is now increasing among African Americans.[26]

Education, again, is the key to avoiding contracting HIV/AIDS. That, and caring people who make every effort to reach at-risk people *before* they contract the virus. Who's at-risk besides homosexuals? African Americans, intravenous drug users, rural populations, urban populations, Caucasians, heterosexuals, Hispanics. Teens are especially at risk because many begin risky behaviors such as unprotected sex and using tainted needles. Drugs and alcohol by themselves are risky for teens.

When you combine either one with sex, the chances of using a condom decreases and the risk of HIV and other infections increases. That "party" can cost them their lives.

Fortunately, there is evaluated curriculum that works. The Centers for Disease Control has evaluated curricula in sexuality education and HIV/AIDS prevention. Two units that have proven successful on a number of criteria are *Get Real About AIDS (GRAA)* and *Becoming a Responsible Teen (BART)*.[27] See chapter 8 for more information.

Certainly among adults, not all feel threatened enough to protect themselves. We still see adults smoking even though they may have had pneumonia several times and are short of breath when they climb the stairs. Some adults still have unprotected sex even when they have been tested and found to be HIV positive.

Even the best media campaign won't work in isolation. It has to be part of a full scale societal force involving federal and local governments, schools, churches, non-governmental agencies, community groups, clinics, parents, and teens. Ideally, everyone would buy into "Safer Sex or No Sex," and accept the fact that teen sex does happen. If and when it does, teens need to be respectful and responsible by practicing safer sex. They will not be frowned upon for having sex, but they will certainly be frowned upon for having unprotected sex. To be absolutely safe, practice abstinence. For safer sex, use condoms and a female contraceptive. For unsafe sex, use neither.

Or listen to my adult granddaughter, Rebecca: "Grandma, your generation worried about getting pregnant. *We worry about dying.*"

Do Condoms
Belong in Schools?

*I was brought up Catholic and went to Catholic School
for eight years. It was strict; we were taught abstinence
only, and even that was only occasionally. My parents were
very open minded, though, and we discussed everything.
They said I should be married before I had children, but
they also told me about contraception and how to get it. At
the public high school I attended there was lots of sex ed
and a bowl of condoms in the nurse's office. The school
was in a very Catholic area of Canada, but the Church
there had no control over school policies.*

Craig, 24. New Brunswick, Canada

"If you teach sex education, they'll have sex, and if you make
condoms available, they'll use them!" It's a comment often heard
in arguments over sexuality education. The data tell us that the
first part is false and the second part is true. Is this good or bad?
It depends on your point of view.

The data on comprehensive sexuality education continue to show that it is effective. As adolescents become more knowledgeable about their bodies, about conception and contraception, and about the spread of sexually transmitted infections, the following results occur: they initiate sex later, and they are more likely to use protection when they do become sexually active.

Importance of Easy Access

Even for those teens who are aware of methods, services, where to obtain them in confidence, and who have overcome embarrassment, barriers remain. These include cost, time constraints, lack of insurance, long waits, inaccessible locations, lack of transportation, and inflexible operating hours. Missing are the very ingredients that make reproductive services work in countries like the Netherlands, France, and Germany — specialized staff training in adolescent development and positive staff attitudes toward patients. Europe has managed to demedicalize reproductive services, and in so doing, to humanize them. Compare their statistics with ours (page 47) to see how well their system works.

In the United States difficulty of access is often cited as a reason for inconsistent use of condoms. Condoms are not easy to get. Unlike the Netherlands, where condom machines can be found side by side with cigarette machines, and where they are in nearly all men's and women's public restrooms, teens here have to look hard for them.

I saw condom machines in nearly every women's restroom I visited in Europe; I didn't see one in the United States until August, 1998. It surprised me in a gas station in Elkton, Virginia. Two kinds were available at 75 cents each, with a disclaimer, "Not guaranteed to be 100 percent effective."

True, we have drugstores and we have clinics, but far too few of the latter. If there is a clinic, the hours may be incompatible with teen school and work schedules, and at a location requiring transportation. We have some schools where teens can get condoms in the nurse's office.

Condoms need to be available beyond schools and clinics. They need to be as available as CDs or chewing gum. Teens (and adults) need to be able to find condoms in clinics, gas stations, airports, restaurants, teen hangouts, work places, restrooms, bars, beauty shops, colleges and universities. Parents could have them at home, in a place where teens can access them in privacy.

Midge Ransom, health educator, talked about the father who lives in a small town in Kansas. To his dismay, his town chose not to participate in a county teen risk-reduction program. As his part in reducing sexual risks for teens, he regularly places bowls of condoms in beauty shops, restaurants, and other places where teens congregate.

Ransom also described the Brown Bag approach followed by the Health Department in Ottawa, Kansas. Cards are passed out with the message, "Respect Yourself, Protect Yourself," and, on the other side, "Bag It! Condoms available. Ask for a brown bag." Each brown bag contains several condoms. Being able to request condoms without saying the word is sometimes important, even for adults, she commented.

Question of Condoms

We can offer sexuality education without fear of students initiating earlier sex. We can also make condoms accessible, assuring ourselves that when they do have sex they will be protected against pregnancy, HIV/AIDS, and other sexually transmitted infections. They will also be far less likely to need an abortion. The case for having condoms widely available, including in the schools, is a good one. But what does "making condoms available" really mean?

When I worked in the Brookline, Massachusetts, school system in the eighties, the community was torn apart by the new idea of having a bowl of condoms in the nurse's office. It was at the beginning of the AIDS epidemic, and the arguments in the School Committee room were heated and lengthy. Doctors and researchers cited the data and warned of the future of AIDS. They told parents that they would be responsible for the illness and death of their children if they did not provide this protection.

Priests, ministers, rabbis, and other religious leaders warned of the future of children whose souls would be lost because of the encouragement of teen sex by, of all things, the schools. These were the schools to which they sent their children for education and protection. Although there had been schisms in the political realm for some time, this was the beginning of the split in the community between the social conservatives and the more liberal thinkers. After months of haranguing on both sides, the more liberal point of view won and condoms were made available in a bowl in the nurse's office.

In 1998, 418 public schools in the U.S. were making condoms available to students.[1] Condoms in some school clinics have become more acceptable over the years, although there are still communities where there is outrage and shock when this type of access is recommended. When the issue is presented as prevention for sexually transmitted infections it is often more palatable to a community than when it is presented as pregnancy prevention, although parents worry about both.

Views on Condom Availability

Teens, according to an informal survey reported by the *Sex, Etc. A Newsletter by Teens for Teens*, approve of condom availability in high schools. Seventy-five percent said schools should make them available and 64 percent said their availability would not encourage them to have sex.

This distribution does not contradict the message that abstinence is best, said 47 percent, but it would reduce teen pregnancy and the spread of STIs (87 percent). Parents should not need to give permission, said 83 percent, and schools should also offer sexual health counseling (62 percent) and teach about how to use condoms (79 percent). While 45 percent said they should be available in the nurse's office, 49 percent opted for machines in the restrooms.[2]

This survey made it clear that teens want condoms, will not abuse them, and if they have sex, most will use them. But it still pointed out that 20 percent of the 59 percent of sexually active teens have never purchased condoms. The disturbing news here is that these students may be having unprotected sex, are not protected from STIs, and possibly are not using any method of birth control. That's a lot of teens to worry about.

The medical profession is worrying about it. The American Academy of Pediatrics, an organization of 49,000 pediatricians, says that while sexual abstinence should be encouraged, youth who want condoms should be able to get them. They feel schools are an appropriate site for their availability. They further state that public health concerns make it necessary to remove barriers and restrictions for condom availability. They base this policy statement on the fact that the United States has the highest teen pregnancy rate of any developed nation and the number of teens with HIV infection doubles every 14 months.[3]

From their medical perspective, they warn that adolescents are far more likely than adults to suffer from infections. Teens are also more likely to suffer lifetime consequences such as chronic infection, ectopic pregnancy, infertility, spontaneous abortions, and infected offspring. They also realize that to be most effective, condom availability should be developed through a collaborative community process. Availability, they add, must be accompanied by school health education programs, parental involvement, counseling, and positive peer support.

In addition to citizen groups that express support and resistance, we find both points of view coming from organized religion. The Anglican Archdeacon Dr. Arnold Hollis of St. James Church, Sandys, England, placed baskets of condoms at the back of his church. He told his congregation that if condoms are not distributed in schools he would ". . . feel that the idealistic Puritanical moralists in our society will be contributing to the genocide of our people."[4] Although he received support from a number of health and educational organizations, he was criticized by others.

Some communities understand the need for collaborative effort. In 1994, San Francisco officials were motivated by an AIDS activist group called ACT-UP and a 1991 school district Youth Behavior Risk Survey that showed students to be at high risk.

The city began a pioneering program to provide free condoms to students in the city's public high schools.[5]

Controversy surrounded the move. A school health advisory committee recommended that a comprehensive sexuality education program be initiated and that free condoms accompany it. In spite of some parental opposition, and after long debate, the proposal was approved and in place by 1993.

The plan as adopted was sensitive to the needs of parents who want to be in full control of the sexuality of their children. One aspect of the Condom Availability Program (CAP) offers parents the opportunity to prohibit their children's eligibility to receive the condoms. Another is that abstinence is stressed as the only 100 percent effective means of prevention of both pregnancy and STIs.

Health organizations, rather than teachers, send volunteers to provide the condoms. Public and private grant funding supports CAP. Data gathered from this program indicate that it is well tolerated in the community, and that students are exhibiting less risk behavior and are not engaging in increased sexual activity. This model appears to be operating relatively smoothly.

School nurses in other districts, on their own, sometimes provide condoms by putting a supply in a discreet place in their offices. They find them gone and never know who took them.

When I spoke with a school nurse in Maine who provides condoms in this way, I asked her how she was preparing her own boys, now 15 and 11.

"We talk about postponing relationships simply because life is complicated enough without girls, and that you should be married when you have children," she said.

I asked her if she had instructed her boys about what to do in the event that they do get sexually involved. She said no, she hadn't talked about that. She hadn't seen her elder son in a relationship that looked like he would get involved. She thought he was more interested in sports than in girls.

I asked her if he knew how to access and use contraception if he did get involved, and she said she wasn't sure. I told her about Stephanie, who, rather than disappointing her mother by asking for help in obtaining contraception, became a teen mother. We talked about the difference between a teen coming to his mother and knowing how to access contraception and information on his own.

Unknown to her, her sons were listening to her end of the conversation. After she hung up they began to talk to her in earnest about their issues concerning sexuality. She wrote me a note:

"Ev, it looks like the boys and I are really going to talk."

Students Take the Lead

Most schools in Maine do not have condoms available even though they offer comprehensive sexuality education. However, students can get information and condoms at family planning clinics, and, if they can find them, in condom machines. When some students were asked if they wanted condoms in nurses' offices, they said they'd prefer to have them in the boys' and girls' restrooms. This they considered genuine access. Any action on their part that involved an adult knowing they wanted a condom was not genuine access, they said.

Sometimes the impetus for condoms in the school comes from the students themselves. Lincoln Academy, in Newcastle, Maine, is one of ten private schools in rural areas in Maine for students who live in nearby school districts that do not have their own high schools. These schools serve public school students, with the communities paying the tuition.

In the fall of 1995, four students from Lincoln Academy attended the Department of Education HIV Prevention Student Leadership Conference where their interest in HIV/AIDS was aroused. With permission from Headmaster Howard E. Ryder and support and encouragement from Sharon G. Morrill, director of the school-based health center, they began exploring the issues. First they worked with an interactive theater group to establish an HIV skit for public presentation.

In the summer of 1996, they tried to go to the AIDS NAMES Project in Washington, DC, but could not get funding. One student went on her own. By the fall of 1996, they had grown to eight members who attended the annual Sugarloaf HIV Prevention Conference. After this conference they decided to focus on condom availability at their school. Needing advice on how to go about doing this, they contacted Advocates for Youth in Washington, DC, for technical assistance.

A year later, in 1997, they heard a Mt. Desert Island High School team present at the Sugarloaf HIV Prevention Conference and began communicating with them. The headmaster allowed them to conduct a school-wide student survey on sexual involvement and attitudes.

Of the 298 returned surveys, only four were opposed to condom availability. At the Sugarloaf Conference in 1998 the students won honorable mention for their work. They were commended for educating the public and their peers in preparation for proposing condom availability at the school. The students then prepared a proposal for the board of trustees. The student council endorsed their proposal.

They then did the necessary political things: surveyed the faculty, conducted a parent focus group, applied for and received a grant to fund the project. They also presented to the superintendent and to a community forum, and held public hearings. There was some community disapproval, support from two local newspapers, and then more public hearings.

In June of 1999 the Board of Trustees voted twelve in favor and four opposed to the installation of two condom vending machines at the school. In August of '99 the two machines were purchased and installed in the boys' and girls' restrooms in the school. It had taken four years of work, but the students had provided genuine access to condoms in their school.

According to Morrill, who is also the health educator, the students learned a lot, not only about STI prevention, but about the politics that surround these issues. They learned how to work with the system, how to win people over to one's point of view, and how to be active citizens in a democracy.

Forty-five percent of the students were sexually active, with 70 percent of this group having had unprotected sex. Fifty-three percent of the sexually active said that with condom availability in the school, they would increase their use of protection. What magnificent success in all ways!

Where Do *You* Stand?

The history of districts and individual schools where condoms have been placed is filled with citizen conflict and hard work on the part of proponents. It's not an easy thing to do. There could also be a dilemma for some in the issue of accessibility. Although anonymous access (i.e. school restrooms) is most desired by teens, and probably most useful, disapproving adults could then say they have no control over their children's access. Even approving adults could be concerned if no counseling is attached to the condom availability program.

Picture this situation, in a comprehensive high school, in a lower middle to upper middle class community. Years before it was all upper middle class white, but now it is almost 50 percent non-English speaking, with pockets of poverty. Many students do not go on to higher education, many continue in technical schools and junior colleges, while some go to four-year colleges and universities.

The question of putting condoms in the nurse's office comes up at a school board meeting. Some members of the board are in favor and some are violently opposed. They reflect the tenor of the community itself, with the full range of feelings. There is some fanatical behavior at the meeting with those on the right calling down the wrath of God and those on the left screaming the statistics on AIDS, other STIs, and teen pregnancy.

You are the principal of the high school and are being asked by both the board and the community to state your point of view. You must take a stand. If you are inclined toward the right you may agree with the religionists. If you are inclined toward the European approach, you are enitrely pragmatic and non-judgmental about teenage sex. If you are a moderate centrist you may see both points of view, *but you must take a stand.*

If you take a stand advocating condoms in the school clinic, you may lose your job. If you don't advocate them, others may protest. Is this a dilemma? Of course. Your work and your income are vital to the well-being of your family.

There is no single answer for all of us. Rather, the power is in the hands of each of us to make the decision we choose and to live with the consequences. If we could mobilize the community to take a stand, perhaps we could convince the school board that they run the risk of not being re-elected if they do not meet the needs of the majority. Then the power might revert to the centrist position of the argument.

We need condom availability in the schools. It appears that they are more accessible from the teen point of view if they are in places where teens can get them anonymously. Yet legislators introduce bills that call for parent approval for teens to access contraception. If we listen to teens, we know that this will lead not to less sex, but to more unprotected sex. The result would be more teens exposing themselves to pregnancy and disease.

The lesson in Maine is clear. Give teens the education to understand the problems. Give them the respect and responsibility they need to view themselves as valuable. Then give them access to contraception should they make the choice to become sexually active before they are ready to become parents. Provide this access especially so they will never become victims of debilitating infection or even death. The statistics in Maine tell the story: one of the lowest teen birth rates in the country and one of the lowest sexually transmitted disease rates as well.

We need to give our young people the resources to protect themselves. As part of the campaign to make condoms widely accessible to all ages, support the schools as an appropriate location for adolescent access. *Condoms need to be widely available, and schools are a logical location for adolescents.*

CHAPTER

12

Nobody *Likes* Abortion

I was pregnant at 13, and I figure that my parents or my older sister who also got pregnant at 13, should have educated all the rest of us after her mistake. But they didn't. We both had abortions. I remember being scared and not knowing what was going to happen. It was hard not being able to express myself to my parents.

My mother took me for the abortion, then had me go to the doctor to get put on the pill. I had no choice about the pill. My mother put me on it because she'd rather have me do that than talk to me about sex. But even then I wasn't careful about disease and we never talked about it at home or at school. I feel lucky I made it through without getting sick.

Abbe, 38, Maine

Just say the word — abortion — and people get emotional. Affecting adult women as well as teens, this issue evokes passion. People of opposing views dig in their heels, insisting that they are right and that those who don't agree with them are wrong.

While they see the issues that divide them, they often don't realize how much agreement there is between the two factions. *No one likes* abortion. *No one* wants young teens to get pregnant or become teenage parents. *No one* wants to see unwanted children brought into the world. *All of us* want to lower the abortion rates.

But there are real disagreements as well. On one side is the view that unmarried teen sex, abortion, *and* the use of contraceptives are immoral, the position of many pro-life advocates. The other view, commonly termed pro-choice, is that unprotected sex is unsafe and irresponsible, and bringing unwanted, unplanned children into the world is immoral. Therefore, according to this view, denying teens access to contraception and to abortion is also immoral.

This battle becomes the most dramatic, filled with the most angst, the most hysteria-producing of any of the battles between Right and Left. It provokes even more emotional response than sex education. No skirmish this — this is warring over the most intensely held beliefs of the human spirit. So powerful are the arguments, both pro-choice and pro-life, that people are killed in the name of saving lives.

Just as the Crusaders chopped off heads of "non-believers" and impaled them on stakes in the name of a loving God, so do modern day pro-life crusaders maim and kill abortion providers in the name of saving lives. Pro-choice advocates, though not given to physical violence, fight with all the other weapons at their command — the media, marches, lobbying, and voting.

Strong Emotions in Abortion Arena

What causes this tremendous emotional outpouring? Any issue that deals with life or death brings out our deepest values. We get exercised about euthanasia in the same way. Abortion causes even more intensity because it is also tied up with sex.

Many pro-choice supporters believe that sex is a private act, a personal act, one that may be pleasurable and recreational in addition to being procreational. Some pro-lifers believe that sex is a part of marriage, and was given to us by God for procreational purposes only.

These views about sex spill over into our views about conception, contraception and abortion. And why not? We're dealing with sex, God, life, death, morality, power, and America's most heartfelt value, freedom. How could we not be emotional when two of our most revered documents, the Bible and the Constitution, are in conflict?

Should conception be viewed as a natural result of the sex act? In the reproductive system a sperm meets an egg and together they form an embryo; in the digestive system food is ingested, digested, and eliminated. Both of these functions are accomplished according to the built-in abilities of the body to perform these functions of life. Or should conception be viewed as an act of God, the giving of life that begins at conception? In the view of pro-choice advocates, an embryo is aborted. In the view of pro-life advocates, the abortionist and the potential mother have committed murder.

So we are not talking about which movie to see, or which candidate to vote for — we're talking about matters of morality, values, ethics, life and death. The pro-choice advocate says: my morality means we have to think of the physical and emotional health and welfare of the mother as well as that of a potential child. If the parents are not ready for a child, either because of the timing, their financial situation, the state of the relationship between the partners, family problems, their ages, a child should not be brought into the world, unwanted. Is this not an immoral thing to do?

The pro-life advocate says none of these issues matter. Their morality says a baby has been conceived and it is God's will that it be born. Let the birthparents place their child for adoption. Someone else will want it. But, for the sake of God, and for your immortal soul, do not murder it.

Pretty powerful arguments on both sides, and pretty emotional. That's why it's an argument fraught with such a potential for violence. Never mind that lives may be taken in the heat of battle — the end justifies the means.

The Facts on Abortion

What are the statistics on abortion in the United States today? The facts:

- Between 1990 and 1996 the number of abortions per year fell from 1.61 million to 1.36 million.[1]
- The rate fell 16 percent, from 27.4 per thousand women to 22.9.[2]
- An estimated 43 percent of women will have at least one abortion by the time they are 45.[3]
- 55 percent of abortions are to women under 25, including 33 percent to women aged 20-24, and 22 percent to teenagers.[4]
- Caucasian women account for 61 percent of all abortions.[5]
- African American women are nearly 3 times as likely as Caucasian women to have an abortion.[6]
- Hispanic women are twice as likely.[7]
- Women who report no religious affiliation are four times more likely to have an abortion than those who report some affiliation.[8]
- Catholics are 29 percent more likely to have abortions than are Protestants.[9]
- One-third of abortions are obtained by married women.[10]
- 15,000 reported abortions are the result of rape or incest.[11]
- 57 percent of the 6.4 million pregnancies each year are unplanned. Of this percentage 53 percent occur in the 10 percent of fertile women who do not practice contraception.[12]
- 88 percent of abortions occur within the first trimester, and only 1.3 percent after 21 weeks.[13]

What does all this mean? What are the trends? First, we see that after a rise during the 1980s, the rate of abortion has been declining. Still, the rates are high compared with other developed countries. Contrary to the public image, we also see that Caucasian women have the majority of abortions in the U.S. However, African American and Hispanic women are more likely to have abortions. It is heartening for those who believe in the value of contraception that we are seeing a downward trend in abortion. It is also heartening for those who believe in the value of religion that women with religious affiliations are less likely to have abortions.

It is disheartening that the ten percent of fertile women who do not use contraception are responsible for over half of the abortions, and that there are still many abortions among women who use contraception and who have religious affiliations. Why?

Of the women who use contraception, six out of ten having an abortion report contraceptive failure.[14] One problem may be the lack of information about the efficacy of the Double Dutch method, i.e. the use of the pill or comparable contraceptive in conjunction with the condom. The Dutch see this as double protection: against pregnancy and against sexually transmitted infections.

The other problem is lack of education concerning the use of the condom. Women and men, including teenagers, are not taught the proper method of putting it on and taking it off, thus minimizing its effectiveness.

Unfortunately, in many areas of the country, these statistics and this information are either not taught to young people in schools or the information given is not research-based. In their personal zeal to promote abstinence only, or as a response to the political climate in which they are teaching, teachers either do not inform their students at all or misinform them about the efficacy of properly used contraception.

A demographic look at the women who do not practice contraception reveals that this practice is greatest among the unmarried, the poor, the young, African American and Hispanic women.[15] Are they having more sex? Not likely. Just having less access to contraceptives, less managed care coverage, less information concerning their availability and use, less cooperation from their partners, and in some cases a social stigma against the use of contraception. This is also the group that is more likely to turn to abortion.[16] So here we are again — if we want to prevent abortion, we must prevent pregnancy. If we want to prevent pregnancy, we must teach abstinence plus other methods of contraception, not abstinence only.

Government Involvement

What is our government doing about this? Is it helping? Yes and no.

Yes. Publicly funded family planning services (Title X) have prevented an estimated 1.3 million unplanned pregnancies annually. About 632,300 of these pregnancies would probably have terminated in abortion resulting in a 44 percent increase over the current estimate of 1.4 million abortions.[17]

No. Medicaid payment for the abortions of poor women are restricted to cases of rape, incest, or women's life endangerment.[18]

No. In 1996 Congress allocated $250 million for Abstinence-Until-Marriage education. States that accept money from the grants must match $3 for every $4 in federal money. This program, which will cost about half a billion dollars, does not permit mention of any method of birth control beyond abstinence. The federal grant of $250 million to states to teach Abstinence Only is not helping prevent pregnancy, infections, or abortion.

No. Many states are implementing laws erecting barriers for young women attempting to obtain reproductive health services, including contraception, ECP (emergency contraceptive pill), or abortion.

Some results of these policies? Poor teen mothers raising unplanned children, often alone, is the first serious result. When I asked one fifteen-year-old if she had considered abortion or adoption when she found out she was pregnant, she said, "No, I never considered adoption. I couldn't consider abortion because it wouldn't be paid for, but the birth expenses would be."

Title X is doing a good job for the young people it reaches. Other policies at the federal level, and more frequently now at the state level, are counter-productive to the goal of limiting the number of abortions.

How did we get to this confusing mix of policy? A short history[19] of abortion law in this country will help us figure out what is happening now:

- Abortion was permitted by common law at the signing of the Declaration of Independence and the U.S. Constitution.

- Abortion became illegal in the middle of the nineteenth century to protect the health of mothers from dangerous patent medicines sold as abortifacients.

- By 1900 abortion was illegal throughout the United States.

- In the 1960s state legislatures, pressured by public opinion and medical, legal, religious, and social welfare organizations, began to reconsider the issue.

- During this period when abortion was illegal, between 200,000 and 1.2 million women obtained illegal abortions annually, and many died.

- Between 1967 and 1973, 17 states reformed anti-abortion laws or repealed them.

- In 1973 the Supreme Court Decision, Roe v. Wade, made abortion legal in the United States. This decision held that a woman had the right to choose an abortion as a constitutional, fundamental right to privacy. It also held that this right is not absolute, and must be balanced against the state's legitimate interest in protecting both the health of the woman and the developing human life. This gave the states some rights to regulate abortion. States, however, could not interfere with a woman's right to choose during the first trimester, and could not restrict or prohibit abortion until roughly the end of the second trimester.

- Some states tried to restrict abortions further. Most state attempts to restrict by requiring waiting periods, husband veto, or performance in hospitals only were struck down by the Supreme Court. The Court upheld some requirements for parent involvement and restrictions on public funds providing abortion services.

- In 1989 the Supreme Court changed direction. It now indicated that it might approve a wider range of state imposed restrictions.

- In 1992, in Planned Parenthood v. Casey, the Supreme Court upheld the right to abortion, but the ruling weakened women's and physicians' legal protection. It gave states the right to enact restrictions that do not create an "undue burden" for women seeking abortion.[20]

This is the change that brings us to the place we are now, where states are becoming increasingly active in imposing restrictions, especially on teens, and the Court is increasingly willing to allow them to do so. Proponents of both views, understanding this, are working harder than ever to influence public opinion and law.

We continue to struggle with this issue. Science and medicine often provide us with answers before we know the questions. One such new finding is the medical abortion pill, mifepristone, called RU-486 in Europe. This is a different drug than ECPs. It is used for early abortions in France, Sweden, Great Britain, and China, but has not been approved for distribution in the United States.[21]

Given that so many Americans dislike abortion, this new medical protocol will contribute to the abortion debate. Anti-abortion advocates, drug companies, family planning agencies, politicians, leaders on the religious right, and Congress will all have to work out their differences before this is available to American women.

Loaded Language Fires Debate

What are the weapons of the proponents of these different points of view? They are using the weapons of successful salesmanship. Reach people where they live. Get them in the heart or the brain or even in the gut, but get them to react. If you can make them react emotionally, that's one way. If not, try reason.

But use any weapon you can find to get public opinion on your side. That's how you make changes in law and education.

Both groups lobby for laws that support their view, they garner support from like-minded organizations, they make appeals to emotions, to rational arguments based on data, to arguments based on theology, and they appeal to values and morality. At their worst, they tell horror stories, circulate misinformation, use fear and intimidation, and ultimately resort to violence.

Horror stories seem to be a popular weapon of the right. Take a specific horror story, move people's emotions, and then generalize from that to either cement their beliefs or to convince them of the rightness of their cause. When you seek to change minds, you know that loaded language is a powerful weapon in a dangerous debate. Are we talking about fetuses or babies? Are we talking about abortion or murder? Are we talking about gynecologists or about abortionists?

Nowhere was language used more effectively than when antichoice proponents, developing a horror story, created the "partial birth abortion." The term refers to a procedure sometimes used in the last trimester of pregnancy.

The Alan Guttmacher *Facts in Brief,* January, 1997,[22] acknowledges that there are few authoritative data on this procedure. The publication contains a report of a study done on the number of late term abortions performed in the United States in 1992. Although people differ on the issue of when a fetus is viable, Guttmacher says, "Twenty-three to twenty-four weeks of gestation is generally considered a minimum for viability." The overwhelming majority of abortions take place in the first trimester. Almost 99 percent occur within the first twenty weeks.[23]

The reasons people give for waiting included not realizing how many weeks they had been pregnant, difficulty in arranging for an abortion, and, in the case of teenagers, fear of telling their parents about the pregnancy.[24]

Opponents of Roe v. Wade are using this procedure as a lever to limit abortion rights. Anti-choice activists have termed it "partial birth abortion" and sold the notion with gruesome detail. Although blocked in some courts because the bills were too broadly written, the public relations impact has been great. The bill itself is vague, never describing the procedure, although the public rhetoric does with great effect.

Thus, two goals are accomplished: Legislators who might be swayed into voting for it do not realize that they are limiting not only that procedure, but many types of abortions, including those legalized in Roe v. Wade. Second, the public becomes incensed about abortion in general based on the specifics of one infrequent procedure.

The pro-choice people are equally loud in their objections.[25] Their concern is that their opponents, knowing that the American people are not ready for a reversal of Roe v. Wade, are chipping away at abortion rights, making it ever more difficult for women to obtain legal abortions. President Clinton vetoed a 1997 bill to ban "partial birth" abortions, but this did not deter anti-abortionists. In fact, it strengthened their resolve to find ways around the law. The problem for the pro-choicers was that the bill being offered failed to protect women's health, and was so deliberately vague that it could lead to the banning of all abortion procedures.

Fight to Limit Teen Access

The political Right is very active in lobbying for laws that support their point of view. Their primary purpose is to eliminate Roe v. Wade, the Supreme Court decision that makes abortion legal. Failing that, they chip away at the rights given women under the law, principally the right to access. The favorite target seems to be teenage women, the easiest group to alienate since most can't vote and they have no power. Many pro-lifers work to limit access to contraception and to family planning information, as well as to abortion. These policies appeal to some adults who, having little control over their teenage children, welcome any law that *appears* to give them such control.

Unfortunately, these policies do not accomplish their goal of fewer teenage pregnancies and fewer abortions. Some sexually active adolescents will not seek birth control if they have to inform their parents or have their consent.[26] Yet anti-abortion people continue to work on limiting access. Neither side wins all battles, but few issues go uncontested.

For example, Planned Parenthood of the Rocky Mountains (Colorado) joined with the ACLU to challenge a statewide Parental Notification Act which passed by a statewide vote in November of 1998. The law required doctors to notify patients' parents at least 48 hours prior to performing an abortion on girls younger than 18. Planned Parenthood and the ACLU challenged the law because of its "dangerous and unconstitutional nature." Their concern at that time was that it did not contain a judicial bypass clause[27] allowing teens to seek permission from a judge as a possible alternative to involving their parents. In April, 2000, the case was still pending.

Internet communication between two Florida women, one an active pro-choice advocate and the other a Democratic Florida legislator, illustrates the emotional pull of this debate. From Linda Miklowitz, May 6, 1999: "Dear Representative Marjorie — I expected to find a Y by your name on CS1598, the Parental Notice bill, but instead there was an N. Thank you so very much. It is a much, much better vote for the welfare of young women . . . I pray that my Sara, who will be 13 in September, never gets pregnant as an unmarried teenage student. If she does and she is too embarrassed to admit it to me, I don't want her to desperately try to self abort or go to some quack because she can't get a safe and legal abortion."

From Representative Marjorie Turnbull of Tallahassee, May 16, 1999 : "Dear Linda — Yes, I voted against the Parental Notification bill this year. As you know I was very torn over this last year, having talked with parents of young women representing a broad base, and finding to my surprise how many supported notification. This year I was going to do likewise (vote Y), but when the proponents would not even accept Elaine Bloom's amendment concerning incest and Elaine broke down on the House floor, something I have never seen her do in her 20 plus years of service, I snapped. I thought there was no way I was going to be a party to such narrow thinking. They were not concerned about young women. They were only concerned about stopping abortion regardless of the consequences."

If a teen does not have access to an abortion in her state, she may seek help in another state. Conservatives are working to prevent this as well. A pro-life group backed a bill by Republican Representative Ros-Lehtinen of Florida to make it a crime to aid in the transport across state lines of a pregnant teen seeking an abortion.[28] This could affect anyone trying to help from a grand-parent to a religious adviser with up to a $100,000 fine and a year in jail.

Only a girl's parent or parents could take her across a state line without fear of penalties. Some girls don't have parents to help them, and many have parents who wouldn't help them in these circumstances. In other words, if the parents won't or can't, the bill makes sure no one else can either. Lots of potential horror stories here.

Having interviewed more than fifty pregnant and parenting teens, I can see situations in which a pregnant teen would be too fearful to talk with her parents about her situation, but could confide in an adviser or a grandparent. Should this girl have to give birth to a baby she obviously didn't want or likely couldn't parent well? The problem really goes well beyond this bill or this issue.

The problem is that we have a society that is uncomfortable with teen sexuality and imposes ever harsher penalties on it. One study found that states with the harshest laws about abortion also have the lowest support for pregnant and parenting mothers. Louisiana imposes the heaviest legal burdens on women request-ing an abortion, and, at the same time, places third lowest in the fifty states in the ten key indicators of child well-being.[29, 30]

The abhorrence of family planning is so strong among some lawmakers that they don't need any help from lobbyists to be obstructionists, even when the issue doesn't affect our country. Congress delayed passage of the national budget bill because of an inclusion in the defense spending section of money for a United Nations program that pays for family planning in China.[31]

What is the motivation of those who make claims to caring about teen welfare but continue to make access to family planning more difficult? They justify their laws requiring parental consent because of their concern that abortion could have a major impact on a woman's psychological and emotional well-being. Yet these same states allow teens to drop out of high school before graduation, and some permit a minor to marry without parental consent. Both are life defining acts. It appears, then, that while espousing teens' welfare, states are actually enacting laws that reflect their socially conservative agenda.

There are some places teens can go for help. Title X, the 1970 federal family planning funding program, supports clinics that provide services to anyone "who needs them without regard to age or marital status." As a result, Title X-supported clinics have always provided confidential services to individuals, including adolescents who request them. This is a key reason why four in ten teenagers who are sexually active and in need of contraceptive services turn to Title X-funded clinics.[32] Here is the kind of clinic we need widely available if we are going to prevent pregnancy, unwanted children, abortion, and sexually transmitted infections.

The Dutch have made free abortion accessible through fourteen government-funded clinics. Parental permission is required for young people under 16, but very few of these young teens seek abortion. The Dutch policies have so educated them that most do not have sexual intercourse before 16, and those who do use contraception. If a young teen requires an abortion and is afraid to ask a parent, a social worker or other trained adult takes the responsibility. Once again, their liberal policies have limited the need for abortion.

Resorting to Violence

If horror stories and lobbying for laws don't work, ultra anti-abortionists go the route of instilling fear, intimidation, and finally resorting to violence. The end result of some of the violent rhetoric is violent action. Dr. Barnett A. Slepian, who worked in a family planning clinic, was a victim of this violence.

While at home with his family, he was assassinated by an extremist sniper with a high powered rifle.[33]

So militant are some of the anti-abortionists that they have created Old West style bounty hunters on a web site that lists the names of abortion providers. The web site is called "The Nuremberg Files" and includes names, addresses, and license plate numbers of medical abortion providers and their families. As they are removed, their names are struck through in red.

Believing that the site intended to continue the violence against such providers, Planned Parenthood sued. A federal jury, hearing the case from Planned Parenthood and a group of doctors who contended that the material amounted to deadly threats, ordered the site to pay more than $107 million to the plaintiffs.[34] The defendants said that nothing in their materials advocated violence, and that their free speech protections had been violated. They vowed to appeal.

This case may well end up in the Supreme Court because of the freedom of speech protection in the Constitution. Still, most people believe this site and others like it are for the specific purpose of stirring up violence against clinics and individuals who provide abortion services. They claim that the deaths of doctors listed on the site, and the greying out of names of doctors injured, attest to the fact that the site, even though not specifically stating it, is symbolically seeking and encouraging violent actions. Supporters say their rights are being trampled. This is an example of the pro-life and pro-choice argument taken to its outermost limits.

Are the anti-abortionists, with their deceptive and violent tactics, succeeding in limiting abortions? There is proof that they are limiting the numbers of clinics. This in itself limits access, especially for poor women without the funds to travel. The Buffalo clinic at which Dr. Slepian worked 23 hours a week, is described as "the only clinic left in Buffalo that specializes in abortions."[35] It vowed to stay open as doctors from all over the country offered their services, and the federal government dispatched marshals to assist clinic workers. Local law enforcement officers, however, did not appear.

The violence and the threats of violence are discouraging others and preventing patients from exercising rights guaranteed by the Supreme Court. For instance, fewer medical schools now train ob-gyn interns in abortion procedures, and fewer physicians are willing to provide abortion services. This is unfortunate for those women who need an abortion.

Fortunately there are legislative responses to these acts of violence.[36] Governor George Pataki of New York proposed legislation to protect women and doctors against violence in family planning/reproductive health clinics after the murder of Dr. Slepian. The new law implying that "New York will not tolerate terrorism" sends a strong message to the extremists.

So did the announcement in Washington by Senator Daniel Patrick Moynihan that any doctor who volunteered to work at that clinic would receive round-the-clock protection from the United States Marshals' Service. Senator Moynihan went on to say that "this was a constitutionally protected medical procedure, and there is a terrorist movement trying to make it impossible."

Continuing the Struggle

With all the problems caused by the fight over abortion, why does it make sense to continue to fight for women's right to privacy and to choice? Some reasons:[37]

- **Legalized abortion is healthier and safer.** The health impact of legal abortion has been examined extensively. Women will seek an abortion whether legal or not. Evidence suggests that practices that permit abortions in proper medical surroundings lead to fewer deaths and complications than restrictive legislation.

- **The public wants legal abortion.** Polls show an over-whelming majority of Americans oppose making abortion illegal again.

- **Legal abortions are done earlier.** Ninety-one percent of all abortions are performed during the first twelve weeks of pregnancy; 96 percent are performed during the first fifteen weeks. Slightly more than one percent are performed past twenty weeks.[38]

- **It is cost effective.** As abortion is prohibited, more public funds are required to pay for maternity care, medical care for the child, and sustenance for the family. For every dollar of public funds that is spent to provide an abortion for low-income women, the expenditure of four dollars in public funds is avoided just in the first two years following birth.

- **It is the responsible and moral thing to do**. Most people, even the most ardent anti-abortionists, would make an exception for the health of the mother, rape, or incest. Many people believe that the emotional and mental health of the mother is equally as important as the quality of life for the child. Teenage parents, trying to raise an unwanted, unplanned child, face too many obstacles to success for themselves and their babies. Even though they may have been irresponsible in conceiving, they deserve a choice about a decision that affects the rest of their lives.

- **If we do not guarantee access, we discriminate against poor women.** Federal legislation such as Medicaid provides medical services to poor women but Medicaid has not paid for abortions since 1976. In many states, poor women have no access. When government gets into the business of prohibiting these rights, it constitutes discrimination against the poor.

- **It is a right guaranteed by the United States Supreme Court.**

Finding Areas of Agreement

As unlikely as it may sound, abortion is another area in which we may come to some agreement. In the Netherlands, France, and Germany, concerned people made social, medical, and religious changes around teen sexuality, not because they wanted more freedom for adolescents, but because of their mutual dislike of abortion. Far from advocating more abortion, though they did advocate the right to abortion, these countries were looking for ways to limit the *need* for abortion. Their goal was to

cut the abortion rates, and to eliminate abortion as a means of
ending unintended pregnancies. They were strongly opposed to
the use of abortion as a method of birth control. Unlike the anti-
abortion activists in this country, they felt the most effective way
to reach their goals was to eliminate unwanted conceptions
through the use of contraception. If the conception never occurs,
the need for abortion never occurs.

In spite of the efforts being made by pro-choice supporters to
provide access to abortion, they agree that our rates of abortion
are too high. They are the highest of the industrialized countries
because we have the highest incidence of unplanned pregnancy,
resulting in a high rate of abortion as well as unplanned births.
While a majority of the public believes we should keep abortion
legal, some object to overuse and others support restricting
access. More effective would be to make abortion less needed by
offering young people the most accessible and friendly contraceptive services available, and combining these services with the
best comprehensive sexuality education possible.

A fitting close for this chapter is a tribute to retired Supreme
Court Justice Harry A. Blackmun, a moderate Midwestern
Republican, who died in November of 1998.[39] During his 24
years on the Supreme Court, he became a passionate defender of
a woman's right to choose abortion. Although he was responsible
for many other important decisions made by the Supreme Court
during his tenure, he knew his legacy would be Roe v. Wade. The
Court found constitutional protection for "a right of personal
privacy that is broad enough to encompass a woman's decision
whether or not to terminate her pregnancy."

The Court fluctuated over the years, but Blackmun held firm
even through his retirement years. He continued to fight for the
right as the Court chipped away at the decision, and as the public
became increasingly vocal about restricting this right.

Fiscally conservative and socially liberal, Justice Blackmun
understood the need for Roe v. Wade, and he fought to retain it
throughout his career on the Supreme Court. Today, as we
continue to fight this battle, we need to elect senators and
representatives with the voice and the soul of Justice Blackmun.

Perhaps one of these will become a Supreme Court Justice.

If we love our children, and we do, and if we care about other human beings, and we do, we can express that love and care by protecting them in whatever way we see fit. Thinking this way, we can defend both the liberal and conservative views that abortion is not a good option by presenting two different routes to prevention: Abstain from sex and you won't need to consider abortion, or contracept carefully and you won't need to consider abortion. *In both cases abortion has been avoided and we have a win/win resolution.*

If our eye is on the prize — reduced abortion — we can reach it from either direction, both based on the ethic of doing good for our fellow human. The solution here is not to limit access as state laws requiring parental notification are trying to do, but to *limit the need.*

13

Attack Problems, Not People

If agreement can be achieved in regard to the values of sexual health, it may be easier to discuss the rules.
Rt. Rev. David E. Richards[1]

The Netherlands, Germany, and France have come to terms with what in the United States is the volatile, value-laden issue of *preventing* teen pregnancy, STIs, and the need for abortion. In the United States, we concentrate instead on abstinence until marriage and intervention services for teenage parents. It's easy to find space in human hearts for innocent babies who need care and protection in spite of their parents' behavior. These European countries have little need for intervention because of their extremely low rates of teen pregnancy, STIs, and abortion. They accept teens' sexual behavior, and they deal with it in a straight-forward, honest, and respectful manner.

This was not always the case. Forty years ago they, too, had conflicting values about teenage sex, unmarried sex, contraception, and abortion, but they resolved their differences for the benefit of their young people. Dr. Evert Ketting of the Netherlands explains, "The so-called 'sexual revolution' was really a moral revolution. This revolution created a new cultural climate in which honesty, openness, frankness, and mutual respect regarding sexuality could flourish. It is my firm belief that this kind of cultural climate is an essential prerequisite for effective prevention of unwanted pregnancy."[2]

Here in the United States, resources, time, energy, expertise, money — all limited and all valuable — are expended on teens and their babies in interventions that range from excellent to poor. Regardless of how good interventions are, they are not preventions. We focus our efforts on intervention; we are scarcely addressing real prevention.

Our hands are tied by conflicting points of view, by arguments being waged, and by decisions either being made that are not win/win or by decisions not being made at all. We need to find areas on which most of us can come to agreement. Then we can begin to make decisions that will bring about a societal change that truly deals with prevention.

Areas of Possible Agreement

We must find ways of communicating that are not prone to blow-ups, name-calling, and angry editorials. Only then can we get on with the business of reducing teen pregnancy, sexually transmitted infections, and abortion.

1. Professional dealmakers say it's good to start with something that's easy to agree on. *There could be agreement that we all want healthy teens.*

2. Since teen pregnancy and sexually transmitted infections contribute to unhealthy lives for teens and their babies, *we could agree that we want to reduce teen pregnancy, HIV/AIDs and other STIs.*

3. Many agree, even the most liberal thinkers among us, that sexual intercourse is not the best choice for young teens. True,

fundamentalists would say it's not moral, it's not appropriate, and it's not permitted, not only for young teens, but for anyone who is not married. However, in a fundamentalist belief system, it would be moral for a young teen to have sex *if* s/he were married. Others would draw the line here and say, "Sex is not a good choice for young teens, nor is early marriage." Even if there would not be agreement about the morality of the issue, *there could be agreement that postponing adolescent sex is an important prevention goal.*

4. We all agree that it's better to prevent an unwanted pregnancy than to need an abortion. The fundamentalists decry it on moral grounds as being against God's will, in fact as murder. They do not believe abortion should be a right; in fact, they think it should be outlawed. Some people say it's not a good thing, not because of the morality issue, but because it can be avoided. If young people, and older people as well, used contraception properly, they could avoid unplanned pregnancies in the first place. They point to the pill, to the condom, to other methods of contraception, and to the morning after pill in the event of human failure or contraceptive failure.

They also believe, that in spite of their dislike of the procedure, abortion must be an accessible choice. Although neither group agrees with the other about the right to abortion or about the morality of the issue, *there could be agreement on the goal of lowering the rate of abortion.*

5. Many people agree that the best thing would be for teens to complete their high school education before getting into sexual relationships that could hinder their personal growth by handicapping them with children or with sexually transmitted infections.

Some groups talk about 18 as being the youngest appropriate age for serious commitments; others say it depends on the maturity and commitment of the young couple; still others say that age is not the defining factor, marriage is. Since marriage in our society rarely takes place before the age of 18, *there could be agreement on the goal of guiding young people toward finishing high school before making a commitment to a relationship that may include having children.*

6. No one, no matter what his or her religious/moral values, objects to inculcating respect and responsibility into young people. *There could be agreement that respect and responsibility be the goals of whatever sexuality education is provided.*

Can we agree on these goals?

• Healthy teens.

• Lowered rates of teen pregnancy.

• Lower rates of HIV/AIDS and other sexually transmitted infections.

• Less need for abortion.

• The postponement of sexual intercourse until teens are old enough to make a commitment to a loving relationship.

• The completion of high school.

• The embedding of the goals of respect and responsibility in all sexuality education.

Agreeing on these goals could create a strong foundation for coming to agreement about the means.

The Netherlands — From Dissent to Agreement

The Dutch policies came about through a series of agreements among dissenting parties, just as we have here. They came into being over a period of forty years in which they discussed all aspects of teen sexuality, and broadened the concept of rights, respect, and responsibility.

As stated in the Preface, by redefining sex as part of the human condition, and by removing the judgmental factor, they said in essence, "People are sexual beings. They will have sex, even if unmarried, and it's our job to help them protect themselves from having abortions. We don't like abortion, even though we acknowledge a woman's right to have one. We will do everything we can to eliminate the need for abortion as much as we can. It's also our job to protect people from having unplanned children and from getting or giving sexually transmitted diseases."

To this end they provided media campaigns that promoted safer sex or no sex, school sexuality education programs, and public, free clinics that provided counseling and contraception. They demedicalized, depoliticized, and dereligionized sexuality, basing their policies on research.

The results? They accomplished each of their three objectives: the lowest teen pregnancy rates, close to the lowest rates of STIs, and one of the lowest rates of abortion in the western industrialized world. Perhaps the most exciting statistic is that their median age for the initiation of sexual intercourse is 17.7 — in spite of (or because of?) the most liberal policies in Europe. Median age for initiation of intercourse in the United States is 16.3.[3]

Young teens in the Netherlands realize that sex is not the fantasy the media claim it to be. They have been exposed to sexuality education from their earliest years, and they don't look upon sex as the magic bullet to adulthood or beauty or power or popularity. They accept it as part of life. It will be there for them when they are ready to make a commitment to another person. In the meantime they are busy growing up.

Most teens under 16 in the Netherlands don't have intercourse. Since there is very little unintended pregnancy, there is very little abortion. Most young women and older women do not have abortions because they have no need. In fact, only 5.7 percent of the pregnancies (all ages) in the Netherlands are unplanned.[4] Compare this with the higher than 50 percent unplanned pregnancy rate in the United States.

Because of the policies, services, and public education campaigns these young people live with, because there is no judgmental overlay, and because sex is treated as a normal part of human life, most teens delay sex until nearly 18. They are not doing this as a moral imperative, but simply because other options are much more attractive to them. Sex has not been fantasized and romanticized as in our culture. They haven't been

sold on sex; they've been sold on respect, responsibility,
and safety.

Sounds simple? No. People in the Netherlands, France, and
Germany told us it wasn't easy, but they did it. They did it
because they cherish their young people. They see them as their
most valuable resource. Their morality was clear. They said,
"Whatever we each think about sex, about marriage, or about
abortion, we know we have to avoid the bad outcomes. We have
done that with our policies."

Societal Change Necessary

As the teen birthrate in the United States continues to drop we
tend to congratulate ourselves, but we are a long way from
solving our problems. Our birthrate per thousand teens aged 15
to 19 is still eight to thirteen times higher than rates in comparable European nations.[5] In spite of our strong economy, the gap
between the very rich and the very poor continues to grow.
Poverty continues to be one of the major problems in the United
States today.

New health issues have accompanied the breakthroughs in
medication and improved survival rates for AIDS patients. AIDS
patients who are living longer have a longer period of time to
infect others if they do not use protection. Other sexually transmitted infections, notably chlamydia and a resurgence of gonorrhea are infecting teens at a higher rate than in earlier years. So
pregnancy and infection are still with us, and protected sex is
more important than ever.

Older men, particularly immature men, continue to seek out
young women. Teen pregnancy refers correctly to teen mothers,
but many of the fathers are older. Advocates for Youth estimates
that among girls who have given birth by the age of 15, 39
percent of the fathers are 20-29 years old.[6] Fifty percent of births
to teens aged 17 or younger were fathered by males aged 20
or older.[7]

The relationship between teenage women and their older
partners is often voluntary, but certainly not always. Society
needs to address the issue of coercive sex by adult men, strength-

ening the laws concerning rape, statutory rape, and child support.

Although the teen birthrate is dropping, the number of teen mothers who are unmarried is rising. This reflects the behavior of adult women. Society must study the reasons for marriage falling into such disfavor. Although many young people have not seen good relationships between cohabiting adults who are not married, they have also been turned off to marriage by their parents' histories of divorce, separation, abandonment, and the complex legal and social problems of dissolving a marriage.

We see the hardships single teen mothers face while raising their children. Perhaps it's time to make marriage look attractive again. The emotional and financial support children need makes two-parent families sound like a better option.

Many single dads don't stay around to support or help raise their children. Maybe they wouldn't stay around even if they were married. But maybe they would. In our new social marketing campaign, as the media and concerned adults teach and learn the values of respect and responsibility, marriage could be made to look attractive. Long term, monogamous commitment could become "cool."

Reaching Out to Fathers

Those of us who work with adolescent mothers and their babies find it easy to attack the men. Where are they? How could they take advantage of these young girls? We may even go so far as to agree with some of the adolescent mothers who say, "Who needs them?" But if we get beyond the emotional response and look at one of the recent studies of young unmarried fathers we find that they may not be as much at fault as we think they are.[8] The data tell us:

- Seventy-five percent are in a romantic relationship with the mother at birth.

- Seventy-two percent contributed money during the pregnancy.

- Eighty-five percent gave financial support to the child.

- The majority saw their young children (aged 0-3) at least once a week.

Given the number of teen mothers we see who are struggling alone, the data may not persuade us. However, it is still in the best interest of the child that we reach out to the father. Children benefit from the emotional and financial support of two parents. Teenagers in particular benefit from having a father in the home as a male role model.

A father and mother serve as an example of a relationship, and the father may serve as a protector of his daughter. Single motherhood is often a precursor of a daughter's single mother-hood as well.

The National Campaign for the Prevention of Teen Pregnancy urges us to integrate a focus on males in efforts to prevent teen pregnancy. We must reinforce behavioral change for young men just as we do for young women. In addition, we have many good reasons to reach out to involve fathers in the upbringing of their children. Some men may not realize how important they are to their children.[9]

Taking Time to Communicate

The technological speed at which society moves these days is affecting relationships. Perhaps we can't do much about the state of overdrive that most of us live in. Many families don't have dinner together anymore, each member heading for the freezer and the microwave when he or she comes in tired and hungry. There isn't a lot of family talk time.

In a class of twenty eighth graders I surveyed in 1992, sixteen said that most evenings they microwaved their dinner and ate alone in front of the TV.

Some fathers and mothers are too busy or too weary at the end of a working day to be den mothers or soccer coaches, and there isn't a lot of interaction with their children. Too many children can't pick up a game of baseball on the neighborhood field because it isn't there, it isn't safe to go there, or because they are too tightly scheduled. Thus they don't interact with their friends in the neighborhood.

It's up to us, the adults who care about them, to make the time to communicate with them. Talk, interest, sharing, showing, caring — these will go a long way toward helping young people improve their self-image and see that life is for interacting with people as well as with technology.

Strengthening Sexuality Education

Sexuality education must continue to be strengthened. School boards and educators are asking, and rightly so, "How do I know if the effort and money I put in will make a real difference?" The Alan Guttmacher Institute reports[10] that 78 percent of the teens who get pregnant say that the pregnancy was unintentional, and that 3 million teens contract a sexually transmitted infection each year.

The National Campaign to Prevent Teen Pregnancy decided that it was time to review the evaluations of "prevention" programs. It set out to learn three things:[11]

- Is there reasonably strong evidence that a program works?

- Is there reasonably strong evidence that it doesn't work?

- Is the evidence so weak or inconsistent that conclusions about impact cannot be reached?

They reviewed the following types of programs: abstinence only, abstinence plus contraception, STI/HIV prevention focus, improving access to contraception, encouraging communication between parent and child concerning sexuality, multiple component programs, and youth development programs.

The results:

- Abstinence Only programs had *no* significant effects on delaying the onset of intercourse

- Some of the comprehensive sexuality education (Abstinence Plus) and STI focus programs delayed the onset of intercourse, reduced the frequency of intercourse or reduced the number of partners, over a control group.

- STI focus programs showed an increase in condom use over controls.

Characteristics of successful programs are those that:

- Have a clear focus on reducing one or more sexual behaviors (i.e. unprotected sex) that lead to pregnancy and STIs.
- Use age-appropriate materials.
- Last long enough to allow participants to complete important activities.
- Provide basic, accurate information.
- Employ methods that involve participants and allow them to personalize the information.
- Include communication skills.
- Have trained teachers.

It is not surprising that AIDS education increases condom use. Ask any group of teens which they fear more, pregnancy or AIDS, and they clearly fear AIDS. "Pregnancy can mess up your life," they say, "but AIDS can kill you."

In a survey I conducted in Maine, October, 1999, I asked 107 teachers and providers of services to pregnant and parenting teens why they thought Maine had such low statistics on teen births. They almost unanimously agreed that it was:

- The delivery of services.
- Comprehensive sexuality education.
- Family planning clinics.
- A supportive legislature that has enacted liberal laws covering teens' access to such services.
- The "small town" feel of many Maine communities in which adults look out for children even if they are not their own.
- The willingness of teen support personnel to work together for the benefit of children rather than protecting their individual turf.

We have the ingredients here. We can reduce our rates just as the Dutch, the Germans, and the French have. Let's spend the money on programs that work.

High Cost of Teen Pregnancy, STIs

For those who would respond to the more pragmatic point of view, the costs to society, let's look at the costs to all of us of teen pregnancy and sexually transmitted infections.[12] By age 13, 20 percent of U.S. teens have already had their first sexual experience. Seventy-four percent of these were involuntary.[13] The average age at which teens become sexually active is 16. Nearly one fourth of the people infected with AIDS are between 20 and 30 years old. Since AIDS has an average incubation period of from 5 to 7 years, many of these young adults were undoubtedly infected with the virus as teens.

And what are the costs to society?[14]

- Because so many teen mothers do not finish high school, they can't get good jobs and are more than twice as likely as other mothers to become dependent on welfare benefits.

- Women who have their first child as teens receive lower wages, accumulate less work experience, and earn less annually than other women — they earn about 50 percent of the income of those who first give birth in their twenties.

- Because of poor prenatal care, their babies are more likely to have health problems at birth. Some low birthrate babies who survive the first year develop life-long disabilities.

- Children born to teenage mothers are more apt to have problems in school. They will need more educational support services than children of older parents.

The costs to taxpayers? Adolescent childbearing costs the taxpayers $6.9 *billion* each year:[15]

- Increased jail expenses of one billion dollars.
- Increased welfare and food stamp benefits of $2.2 billion.
- Increased medical care expenses of $1.5 billion.
- Increased foster care of $.9 billion.
- Loss of tax revenues of $1.3 billion.

Change doesn't come easily. Even when people don't like

what is happening in their lives, they are still resistant to change. We are comfortable with what we know. It's familiar. The unknown is frightening.

"Uncle Ed," a wise mentor on whom I relied when I was starting a new career in my forties, told me, "Ev, think about the fact that every time you solve a problem you create a new one." He's old, I thought. He's afraid of change. He turned out to be right, merely cautioning me to think carefully about the change I was making. Still, it was important to try to solve the problem, and then it was necessary to try to solve the new one.

So I am not saying we can make change without risk. I am saying we *need* to make change since the risks of staying where we are are far greater than the risks we may create. Our society needs to change. We must consider the societal costs, the social costs, and the financial costs of staying where we are. Then we need to plunge in.

We have the knowledge of how to do it. All we need now is the will and the way. Let's join those who are already working hard for young people, put the interest of our children above our personal preferences, *and remember as we engage in dialogue that it's about them, not about us.*

You Can Help —
Ten Points of Action

I can't believe that the United States, where we say we do not want early sex and teen pregnancy, encourages the media to seduce adolescents by showing casual sex with no consequences. I can't believe that a country that says it loves its children allows a whole group of them to become parents by not giving them the knowledge and support they need to make appropriate and safe decisions. I can't believe that a country that thinks of itself as so aware can't hear these children screaming for help. Is it possible that a country that can rally around a football game or a game show on TV can't get itself organized to combat teen pregnancy and sexually transmitted infections?

Sara Sellinger, 76, Sarasota

As an Individual You Can . . .

If you come from industry, and you are an employer, you need to convince the private sector to get involved with young people.

Employers also need to provide young people with summer jobs and internships as they get involved with them. If you are an employee you need to talk with your fellow employees to educate them about these issues.

If you come from education, you have to communicate with everyone who teaches young people. You must educate school committees and communities about the need for comprehensive sexuality education. You need to let them know that good education programs are research-based and have been carefully evaluated.

If you have a religious affiliation, share your ideas about the new morality with clergy and lay people. Be sensitive to personal beliefs and values, and step aside from personal positions in order to concentrate efforts on common interests such as the good health of young people.

If you are a parent, join parent networks that gather to establish safe boundaries for children. If you are a member of such networks, convince the organization to expand into other neighborhoods and into local government.

If you work in social services, it behooves you to lobby hard with everyone who has any influence over the care and nurturing of teens.

If you labor in medicine and public health, you have a chance to influence the delivery of services to teens. You can exert your influence in the establishment of school-based health centers located either in the school or within walking distance.

If you are in government at any level you are in the best position to initiate and pass laws that protect teens by offering them poverty-free lives and healthy reproductive options.

As a Member of a Group You Can . . .

As part of a group you can address all the issues above, but with the added clout of numbers. If you initiate such a group or become a member of one, think of it as a Task Force that will address one or all of the following Ten Points of Action. The success of such discussions will depend on the strength and skill of the leadership.

A good leader will understand that wise negotiations depend on people giving up their entrenched positions in order to concentrate on mutual interests such as the health of young people. The group will focus on results. A wise agreement, drawn up at the conclusion of the negotiations, will satisfy the legitimate interests of each side and will be fair. It will also be durable, and will take community interests into account. Everyone will feel like a winner.[1]

1. Poverty

Poverty may be the most negative influence in the life of a young person. When parents are struggling to provide the basic necessities of food and shelter there isn't a lot of energy or time left for other kinds of nurture. They have neither the time nor the motivation to provide a stimulating, safe environment. Yes, there are cases in which young people have overcome the barriers of poverty to become happy, successful adults, sometimes emerging even stronger than children of the affluent. To prove this we point to famous personalities who came from ghettos of poverty, but they are the exceptions, not the rule.

For most people, poverty is not a motivator. It does more harm than good with its accompanying joblessness, hopelessness, and sometimes homelessness that result in poor, sick, uneducated, unprepared adults. Poverty breaks up families or keeps new families from staying together. A redistribution of wealth through fairer taxation and minimum wage laws can reduce poverty in America. This is a problem that good people everywhere can recognize and wish it were otherwise, but government must be involved in tackling and solving it. *It's up to us to lobby for legislation and policies that will help to alleviate poverty, especially for families with children.*

2. Parents and Other Mentors

Parents remain the most influential of all, in spite of some belief to the contrary. Loving, listening role modeling parents can establish the behavioral expectations for their children. Even though they think they may not be heard by their teens, they learn later that indeed they were.

Parent networks, successful in local communities, must be expanded. When parents work together to agree on limits and present a united front, it's easier for them to resist the complaint, "Nancy's mother lets her stay out until midnight!" When young people realize that many parents are caring about their well-being, they are likely to feel more protected and less singled out.

Other adults who touch youth through religious organizations, lay organizations, volunteer social or community groups, sports teams, or academic endeavors make a huge difference in the lives they reach. As role models or as interested friends they can provide the lifeline many young people are missing.

Here individuals can make a big difference. Walking, hiking, fishing, and talking with youth are ways to slow down the pace and make stronger connections. *It's up to parents and other adults to provide the time for reflection and connection that teens need to round out their personalities and characters.*

3. The Media

The potential for influence here is limited only by the intent of the media providers. I have spent considerable time and print in this book castigating the media for their obsession with sex and violence and the omission of respect and responsibility from their messages. If they could take all of their creative energy and turn it into positive messages — safer sex or no sex, respect for yourself and your partner, be responsible to yourself, your partner, your parents, and your society — they would become allies in our efforts to raise healthy children.

Government, parents, young people, and the media can form a partnership in which government funds, media, teens and parents plan. Together they could deliver a Safer Sex or No Sex campaign such as that embraced by the Netherlands, France, and Germany. The ads need to be constant, consistent, honest, and teen-friendly. They need to become so much a part of the lives of teens in our society that sexuality education in schools is simply a continuation of the lessons young people have already learned when they come to school. *Our pressure on the media to become a positive force could go a long way toward making it happen.*

4. General Education

Teachers know that grown students who come back to visit, frequently parents themselves, are often the students who were most difficult to teach. Quality education pays off. *We need to lobby for small classes and competitive teacher salaries to attract the best people. We need to vote for qualified school board members who will promote education that will produce knowledgeable, responsible, creative adults.*

5. Sexuality Education

Comprehensive sexuality education (including teaching about abstinence and other methods of contraception, A+) can guide teens into positive, safe relationships just as it has in Europe. Too late or too narrow education can miss the "teachable moments" so that its potential influence is negated by more powerful influences in young lives. *We need to let school boards, local, state, and federal governments know that we support comprehensive sexuality education.*

6. Religion

Conflicts between and among religious organizations use up the energy and resources we need to work for the benefit of our young people. Arnold Burron[2] suggests that one of the tenets of traditionalists is, "Approaches that do not have a clearly defined scope and sequence . . . lead to nebulous goals and subjective outcomes." Burron was referring to outcome-based education in schools, but the insight derived from this statement has relevance to the new morality approach to sexuality education as well.

Traditionalists are seeking clarity and assurance in their lives. Proponents of the European approach to teen sexuality are seeking clearly established values as well. With established rules there is little need for soul searching. If respect and responsibility for safer sex became the rule for all, we would all be at ease. People of all ages would have the assurance that their behavior met their own needs as well as the standards of society. We would all be more secure.

7. Family Planning Clinics

Either in schools or in proximity to neighborhoods, clinics that are accessible and teen friendly can help young people manage their lives so that they grow up strong and healthy, unencumbered by unwanted, unplanned children or by debilitating infection.

Local health departments need to give careful thought to their location. Teens would find it easy to use their services if they were adjacent to schools or located in malls where young people congregate. Often teens don't have transportation so locations within walking distance are a must. *Our voices must be added to those of public health personnel who advocate for such clinics.*

8. Peer Pressure

Peers can be either a good influence or a bad one. Parents, knowing this well, lament the "bad" friends their children love and suggest the "good" friends their children are sure to hate. The Netherlands solved this problem by making respect and responsibility the norm for teen behavior, turning peer pressure into a positive partnership with parents. *Support every effort to bring about this change in our society and teens will become your strongest ally.*

9. Youth Development Programs

Youth development programs that provide motivation to delay intercourse or to contracept carefully have proven effective for teens. These involve mentoring, sports, extra-curricular activities in schools and neighborhood agencies, communication skills, goal setting, and career counseling and interning. There are many roles here for parents and other interested adults. *Vote for such programs with your feet (by attending meetings and signifying your support) and with your pocketbook (by indicating your willingness to pay for them).*

10. Government Policy

In the final analysis it's up to us, the adults, to lobby our government for the support and changes it can effect. Make your votes count. Elect the officials who want the new morality, safer sex or no sex. *Elect the people who will assure that your children and grandchildren will grow up in an environment that is supportive, loving, and healthy.*

Expressing Our Morality

To do this job — raising healthy teens rather than raising babies of teens — we have to suspend our judgmental attitudes, our deeply held moral codes, and exchange them for the new morality. Safer sex or no sex *is* the moral way to go. We love our children, we do not want them to be sick or to die, and we want them to have their own childhoods before they have children.

We can express our morality by depoliticizing the issues of prevention, and by making sexuality a health issue based on scientific principles rather than a political issue. We can all become mentors, we can all become educators, we can all become advocates for teens.

When we choose to get involved, we have a big job to do. As mentors to teens, as their educators, and as good citizens, we have to enlist the aid of every person we meet. We have to lobby the legislators for quality sexuality education and for quality education in every area. We have to sell people on the idea of society valuing young people. We must send the pervasive and consistent message to them that has been so successful in the Netherlands, Germany, and France — be respectful, be responsible, be safe. Perhaps then we can give up the dubious distinction of being number one with the highest teen birth rates, the highest rate of STIs, and the highest rate of abortion of any developed country — and where teens initiate sexual intercourse one to two years earlier than in other industrialized countries.

We know we can mobilize our society when we decide to do it. "Many adults and teens in our society now are either abstinent or are effective contraceptors. Small family size proves that. It's time we brought more young people on board," says Professor Linda Berne, University of North Carolina at Charlotte.

The media can capture the imagination of the whole country on the issue of teen sexuality. Schools *can* lead the way with quality, comprehensive sexuality education. The government *can* fund the media, comprehensive sexuality education, and the clinics. The non-governmental agencies *can* continue their work with teens, and parents *can* become the first educators and mentors. The major issue is the *will* to do it.

Then, teens who are not responsible, who spread disease, or who become pregnant by accident, will know they face the disapproval of their peers and their mentors because they had everything at their disposal to prevent these outcomes. The phrase "safer sex or no sex" can become part of our vocabulary just as "smoke-free" and "designated driver" have.

The new morality would broaden the concept of *abstinence* to mean:

Abstain from early sex if possible.
Abstain from giving or getting sexually transmitted infections.
Abstain from having unplanned babies.
Abstain from the need for an abortion.

The new morality would broaden the concept of *prevention* to mean:

Prevent unprotected sex.
Prevent sexually transmitted infections.
Prevent unplanned pregnancy.
Prevent the need for an abortion.

The message to adolescents is clear. Abstinence is a responsible first choice. If you become sexually active, *Safer Sex,* keeping yourself and your partner safe, is the only respectful, responsible choice.

Think of societal change as a series of ever widening concentric circles. You are in the middle of the smallest circle. As you reach out to family and friends with your message of *The New Morality,* you create wider circles. As they hear you and spread the word further, the circles get wider and wider. *Soon all of us are encircled, focused on the changes needed to protect our most precious resource, our children.*

APPENDIX

RESEARCH CITATIONS

Introduction
1. Cohen, Mark Nathan. *The Culture of Intolerance*. New Haven: Yale University Press, 1998, pp. 62-63.
2. Ibid., p. 139.

Chapter 1. From Prudery to Pragmatism
1. "Teen Sex and Pregnancy." New York and Washington DC: Alan Guttmacher Institute, *Facts in Brief*, May, 1998.
2. *Sex and America's Teenagers*. New York and Washington DC: Alan Guttmacher Institute, 1994, p. 45.
3. Alford, Sue, and Ammie Feijoo. "Adolescent Sexual Health in Europe and the U.S. — Why the Difference?" Washington DC: Advocates for Youth, February, 2000.
4. Brunner, Borgna, editor. *Time Almanac 2000 with Information Please*. Boston MA: Time, Inc., Home Entertainment, 1999.
5. O'Hare, William P., editor. *When Teens Have Sex: Issues and Trends*. Baltimore MD: The Annie E. Casey Foundation, 1998, pp. 56-133.

6. Ibid.
7. Brunner, op. cit.
8. Moore, Kristin A., et al. "The Child Indicator, #642." Washington DC: Child Trends, 1999, p. 3.
9. Brunner, op. cit.
10. O'Hare, op. cit.
11. Males, Mike A. *The Scapegoat Generation: America's War on Adolescents.* Monroe ME: Common Courage Press, 1996. pp. 274-75.
12. Solomon-Fears, Carmen. "Welfare Reform: Provisions Related to Non-marital Births." Washington DC: Congressional Research Service, The Library of Congress, *CRS Report*, June 21, 1999, p. 3.
13. Males, op. cit., pp. 277-78.
14. Ibid., p. 280
15. Ibid., p. 279
16. Berne, Linda, and Barbara Huberman. *Aimer Sans Peur: European Approaches to Adolescent Sexual Behavior and Responsibility.* Washington DC: Advocates for Youth, 1999, pp. 69-70.

Chapter 2. The Struggle for Family Values

1. Guyer, Paul, editor. *Groundwork of the Metaphysics of Morality: Critical Essays.* New York: Roman and Littlefield, 1998, p. XI.
2. Ibid.
3. Sartorius, Rolf. *Individual Conduct and Social Norms.* Encino CA: Dickinson, 1975, pp. 21, 29.
4. Ibid.

Chapter 3. Teen Sex — What's a Parent to Do?

1. Miller, Brent C. "A Research Synthesis of Family Influences on Adolescent Pregnancy." Washington DC: National Campaign to Prevent Teen Pregnancy, April, 1998.
2. Blum, Robert W., and Peggy M. Rinehart. "Protecting Adolescents from Harm: Findings from the National Longitudinal Study of Adolescent Health." *Journal of the American Medical Association (JAMA),* September, 1997.
3. *Sex and America's Teenagers.* New York and Washington DC: Alan Guttmacher Institute, 1994, p. 9.
4. "Ten Tips for Parents to Help Their Children Avoid Teen Pregnancy." Washington DC: National Campaign to Prevent Teen Pregnancy, 1998.

Chapter 4. Influenced by the Media

1. Berne, Linda, and Barbara Huberman. *Aimer Sans Peur: European Approaches to Adolescent Sexual Behavior and Responsibility.* Washington DC: Advocates for Youth, 1999, p. 67.
2. Kunkel, Dale et al. "Sex on TV." Menlo Park CA: Kaiser Family Foundation, February, 1999, pp. 4, 53-55.
3. Sterngold, James. "Lessons Not Quite Ready For Prime Time." New York: *New York Times*, March 28, 1999, p. 5.
4. *Documenting the Power of Entertainment Television: The Impact of a Brief Health Message in One of TV's Most Popular Dramas.* Menlo Park CA: Henry J. Kaiser Family Foundation, 1997.
5. Handelman, Jay. "Let's Talk About Sex and Cancer." Sarasota FL: *Sarasota Herald-Tribune*, September 22, 1998, p. E1.
6. De Jong, William and Jay A. Winsten. *The Media and the Message: Lessons Learned From Past Public Service Campaigns.* Washington DC: National Campaign to Prevent Teen Pregnancy, February, 1998, p. 1.
7. Ibid.
8. Folb, Kate. "A Report from The Media Project." Washington DC: Advocates for Youth, 1999.
9. Rimel, Rebecca W. "A Power to Motivate or Manipulate." New York: *New York Times*, February 14, 1999, Section 4, p. 7.
10. Jamieson, Kathleen Hall. ". . . and Now for Some Good News." Washington DC: *AARP News,* October, 1998, pp.18-19.

Chapter 5. Evolving Role of Religion

1. "Nine Tips to Help Faith Leaders and Their Communities Address Teen Pregnancy." Washington DC: National Campaign to Prevent Teen Pregnancy, 1998.
2. Haffner, Debra W. *A Time to Speak: Faith Communities and Sexuality Education.* New York and Washington DC: SIECUS, 1998, p. 3.
3. Ibid., pp. 7-8.
4. Clarity, James F. "Scandals and New Beliefs Changing Ireland's Church." New York: *New York Times*, June 13, 1999, p. 6.
5. Dillon, Sam. "Smaller Families To Bring Big Change in Mexico." New York: *New York Times*, June 8, 1999, p. 1.
6. Niebuhr, Gustav. "Methodist Leaders Must Weigh Penalties." New York: *New York Times*, June 11, 1999, p. A18.
7. Rosin, Hanna. "Rabbi Group Sanctions Gay Unions." Sarasota FL: *Sarasota Herald-Tribune,* March 30, 2000, p. 1.

8. Maganini, Steven, Andy Furillo, and Ralph Montano. "Three Synagogues Struck by Arson." Sacramento CA: *Sacramento Bee*, June 19, 1999, p. 1.
9. "Nine Tips . . . ," op. cit.
10. Haffner, Debra, and James Wagoner. "Vast Majority of Americans Support Sexuality Education." Washington DC: SIECUS, *SIECUS Report*, August/September, 1999.
11. Gibb, Sarah, editor. *The Advocacy Manual for Sexuality Education, Health and Justice: Resources for Communities of Faith.* Boston MA: Unitarian Universalist Association and United Church Board for Homeland Ministries, 1999.
12. Richards, David E. "Values and Sexual Health." New York and Washington DC: SIECUS, *SIECUS Report*, Vol. 18, #6, August/September,1990.

Chapter 6. Sexuality Education Is Everywhere

1. Brody, Jane E. "Teenagers and Sex: Younger and More at Risk." New York: *New York Times*, September 15, 1998, p. B15.
2. Sadik, Nafis. "United Nations Population Fund Report." Washington DC: Advocates for Youth, November 16, 1998.
3. "Who We Are." New Brunswick NJ: Network for Family Life Education, Rutgers, The State University of New Jersey, www.sxetc.org, February, 1999.
4. Davis, Laura. "Adolescent Pregnancy and Childbearing." Washington DC: Advocates for Youth, *The Facts,* March, 1996.

Chapter 7. Abstinence Only vs. Abstinence Plus

1. "Abstinence Education Programs in Fiscal Year 1998." New York and Washington DC: SIECUS, 1999.
2. Haffner, Debra, and James Wagoner. "Vast Majority of Americans Support Sexuality Education." Washington DC: SIECUS, *SIECUS Report,* August/September, 1999.
3. "Abstinence Education . . .," op. cit.
4. Napier, Kristine. *The Power of Abstinence.* New York: Avon Books, 1996.
5. Hatcher, Robert A., et al. *Managing Contraception.* Tiger GA: Bridging the Gap Foundation, 1999, p. 48.
6. Levenberg, Wrenn, compiler. "Adolescents and Abstinence." Washington DC: Advocates for Youth, *The Facts,* September, 1998.

7. Ibid.

8. *Sex and America's Teenagers.* New York and Washington DC: Alan Guttmacher Institute, 1994, p. 28.

9. Levenberg, op. cit.

10. Hoffman, Anna. "Effective Comprehensive Sexuality Education." Washington DC: Advocates for Youth. *Programs at a Glance,* July, 1997.

11. Herdman, Cristina S. "Promising Adolescent Pregnancy Prevention Programs." Washington DC: Advocates for Youth, *Programs at a Glance,* 1996.

12. "From Research to Classroom." Atlanta GA: Centers for Disease Control and Prevention, *Programs that Work.*

13. Haffner and Wagoner, op. cit.

14. Feijoo, Ammie N. *Teenage Pregnancy, The Case for Prevention.* Second Edition. Washington DC: Advocates for Youth, 1999, pp. 2, 3.

Chapter 8. Sexuality Education — What's a School to Do?

1. Haffner, Debra, and James Wagoner. "Vast Majority of Americans Support Sexuality Education." Washington DC: SIECUS, *SIECUS Report,* August/September, 1999.

2. MacNamara, Marina, compiler. "Sexuality Education Curricula and Programs." Washington DC: Advocates for Youth, *The Facts,* September, 1997, p.1.

3. Berne, Linda, and Barbara Huberman. *Aimer Sans Peur: European Approaches to Adolescent Sexual Behavior and Responsibility.* Washington DC: Advocates for Youth, 1999, p.1.

4. *Life Management Skills.* Sarasota FL: Sarasota Public Schools, 1998.

5. Stevens, Jennifer, compiler. "Peer Education: Promoting Healthy Behaviors." Washington DC: Advocates for Youth, *The Facts,* October, 1996, p.1.

6. Norman, Jane, compiler. "Evaluated Peer Health Education Programs." Washington DC: Advocates for Youth, *Programs at a Glance,* November, 1999, p. 3.

7. Harris, Robie H. *It's Perfectly Normal: Changing Bodies, Growing Up, Sex and Sexual Health.* Cambridge MA: Candlewick Press, 1994.

8. Brick, Peggy, et al. *The New Teaching Safer Sex.* New Brunswick

NJ: Center for Family Life Education, Planned Parenthood of
Greater New Jersey, 1998.

9. Herdman, Cristina S. "Promising Adolescent Pregnancy Prevention
Programs." Washington DC: Advocates for Youth, *Programs at a
Glance,* 1996.

10. Casparian, Elizabeth, Eva Goldfarb, Richard Kimball, Barbara
Sprung, and Pamela M. Wilson. *Our Whole Lives: Comprehensive
Sexuality Education.* Boston MA: Unitarian Universalist Association and United Church Board for Homeland Ministries,
1999-2000.

11. Brownlee, Patricia, et al. Video, "Considering Your Options."
Washington DC: National Education Association Health Information Network, 1998.

12. "From Research to Classroom: Programs that Work."
Atlanta GA: Centers for Disease Control and Prevention.

13. "Appraising Teen Magazines." New Brunswick NJ: Network for
Family Life Education, Rutgers, The State University of New
Jersey, *Family Life Matters,* Spring, 1998, p. 3.

14. Saewyc, Elizabeth M., Linda H. Bearinger, Robert W. Blum and
Michael D. Resnick. "Sexual Intercourse, Abuse and Pregnancy
Among Adolescent Women: Does Sexual Orientation Make a
Difference?" New York: Alan Guttmacher Institute, *Family
Planning Perspectives,* Volume 31, Number 3, May/June 1999, pp.
127-131.

15. Wasserman, Marie. *Learning About Family Life.* New Brunswick
NJ: Network for Family Life Education, Rutgers, The State
University of New Jersey, 1992.

16. Schurmann, Ann. *Baby Steps: Implementing Family Life Education
in the Early Grades.* New Brunswick NJ: Network for Family Life
Education, Rutgers, The State University of New Jersey, 1997.

17. Rodriguez, Monica, Rebecca Young, Stacie Renfro, Marysol
Asencio, and Debra Haffner. "Teaching Our Teachers to Teach: A
SIECUS Study on Training and Preparation for HIV/AIDS Preven-
tion and Sexuality Education." New York and Washington DC:
SIECUS, *SIECUS Report,* December 1995/January 1996.

Chapter 9. Contraception — "It Just Happened"

1. Berne, Linda, and Barbara Huberman. *Aimer Sans Peur: European
Approaches to Adolescent Sexual Behavior and Responsibility.*
Washington DC: Advocates for Youth, 1999, p. 67.

2. Hatcher, Robert A, et al. *A Pocket Guide to Managing*

Contraception. Tiger GA: Bridging the Gap Foundation, 1999.

3. *Not Just for Girls: The Roles of Boys and Men in Teen Pregnancy Prevention.* Washington DC: National Campaign to Prevent Teen Pregnancy, November, 1997, p. 7.

4. Hatcher, op. cit., p. 19.

5. Ibid., pp. 31-33.

6. Ibid., p. 32.

7. Freedman, Alix M. "Why Teenage Girls Love 'The Shot'; Why Others Aren't So Sure." New York: *Wall Street Journal,* October 14, 1998, p. 1.

8. Ibid.

9. Hatcher, op. cit., p. 112.

10. Ibid.

11. "Contraception, Three Days After." New York: *New York Times,* September 4, 1998, p. A22.

12. Trussell, Dr. James. "Emergency Contraception: It Can Change Our World." New Brunswick NJ: *Family Life Matters, #36,* Winter, 1999, p. 1.

13. "Sex-Sensibility: Emergency Contraception Fact Sheet." Alexandria VA: American Medical Women's Association, November 17, 1999, p. 1.

14. Delbanco, Suzanne F., et al. "Are We Making Progress with Emergency Contraception?" Alexandria VA: *Journal of American Medical Women's Association,* Volume 53, #5, November 17, 1999, p.1.

15. Ellertson, Charlotte, et al. "Should Emergency Contraceptive Pills Be Available Without Prescription?" Alexandria VA: *Journal of American Medical Women's Association,* Volume 53, #5, November 17, 1999, p.1.

16. MacNamara, Marina, compiler. "Adolescent Contraceptive Use." Washington DC: Advocates for Youth, *The Facts,* November, 1997, pp.1-2.

17. Moore, Kristin A., et al. "The Child Indicator, #642." Washington DC: Child Trends, 1999.

18. Feijoo, Ammie N. *Teenage Pregnancy: The Case for Prevention,* Second Edition. Washington DC: Advocates for Youth, 1999, p. 2.

19. "Equity in Prescription Insurance and Contraceptive Coverage Act of 1999." Washington DC: U.S. Congress, S.1200, February 22, 2000.

20. "Contraceptive Services." New York and Washington DC: Alan Guttmacher Institute, *Facts in Brief,* January, 1998.

21. Kearney, Sharon. "Title X Family Planning Program." Washington DC: Congressional Research Service, The Library of Congress, *CRS Report*, October 26, 1998, p. 1.
22. "Contraceptive Services," op. cit.
23. Gressle, Sharon. "Federal Civilian Employees and the FY 1999 Budget." Washington DC: Congressional Research Service, Library of Congress, *CRS Issue Brief,* October 30, 1998.

Chapter 10. HIV, AIDS, and STIs — Alphabet of Pain

1. "STD Q & A." Research Triangle Park NC: American Social Health Association, 1997.
2. "Confronting the Hidden Epidemic." Research Triangle Park NC: American Social Health Association, *Annual Report of ASHA,* 1996-97, p. 1.
3. "STD Q & A," op. cit.
4. Alford, Sue, and Gary Linnen, compilers. "Adolescents, HIV/AIDS and Other STDs." Washington DC: Advocates for Youth, November, 1998, p. 1.
5. "Confronting the Hidden Epidemic . . .," op. cit.
6. Alford, op. cit.
7. Berne, Linda, and Barbara Huberman. *Aimer Sans Peur: European Approaches to Adolescent Sexual Behavior and Responsibility.* Washington DC: Advocates for Youth, 1999, p. 7.
8. "ASHA Resource Guide: Facts to Think About." Research Triangle Park NC: American Social Health Association, August, 1995, p. 1.
9. Clark, Peggy. "Awareness of Sexually Transmitted Diseases: An International Study." Research Triangle Park NC: American Social Health Association, August 27, 1995, pp. 1-11.
10. *Sex and America's Teenagers*, New York and Washington DC: Alan Guttmacher Institute, 1994, p.6.
11. Ibid., p. 7
12. Hoffman, Anna. "Effective Comprehensive Sexuality Education." Washington DC: Advocates for Youth, *Programs at a Glance,* July, 1997, p.1.
13. "Loving Safely: What You Need to Know About STDs." Research Triangle Park NC: American Social Health Association, 1998.
14. "HIV/AIDS Prevention Workshop for Teens." Palo Alto CA: Aids Prevention Program, YWCA Flyer.
15. Brown, L., and R. DiClemente. "Predictors of Condom Use In Sexually Active Adolescents." Palo Alto CA: *Journal of Adolescent*

Health, Volume 13: 1992, pp. 651-657.
16. Di Clemente, R., M. Durbin, et al. "Determinants of Condom Use Among Junior High School Students in a Minority, Inner-City District." Elk Grove, IL: *American Journal of Pediatrics,* 89:197-202, 1992.
17. Kegeles, S., N. Adler, and C. Irwin. "Adolescents and Condoms: The Association of Beliefs with Intentions to Use." *American Journal of Diseases of Children,* 143:911-915, 1989.
18. Ibid.
19. Kegeles, op. cit.
20. "STD Q & A," op. cit.
21. Ibid.
22. Ibrahim, Youssef M. "AIDS is Slashing Africa's Population." New York: *New York Times,* October 28, 1998, p. A3.
23. "Trends in the HIV & AIDS Epidemic." Atlanta GA: Centers for Disease Control and Prevention, October 2, 1998, Section 3, p. 2.
24. Ibid.
25. Ibid.
26. Ibid.
27. "From Research to Classroom: Programs that Work." Atlanta GA: Centers for Disease Control and Prevention.

Chapter 11. Do Condoms Belong in Schools?

1. "School Condom Availability and Condom Use Among Teens." Washington DC: Advocates for Youth, *Transitions,* Vol. 10, #1, September 9, 1998, p. 3.
2. "Teen Thoughts on Condom Distribution." New Brunswick NJ: *Daily News,* Campaign for Children, August 29, 1997, pp. 1-3.
3. "Condom Availability for Youth." Elk Grove IL: *Journal of the American Academy of Pediatrics,* Volume 95, #2, February, 1995, pp. 281-285.
4. Burges, Don. "Archdeacon Calls for Condoms in the Schools." Hamilton Bermuda: *Bermuda Sun,* February 7, 1996.
5. Heilig, Steve. "Free Condoms in San Francisco Schools: Five Years and Running." San Francisco CA: San Francisco Medical Society, June 12, 1999, pp 1-3.

Chapter 12. Nobody *Likes* Abortions.

1. Henshaw, Stanley K. "Abortion Incidence and Services in the U.S. 1995-1996." New York and Washington DC: Alan Guttmacher

Institute, *Family Planning Perspectives,* Vol. 30, #6, November/
December, 1998, p. 264.

2. Ibid.
3. Gold, Rachel Benson. *Abortion and Women's Health.* New York and Washington DC: Alan Guttmacher Institute, 1990.
4. Ibid.
5. "Induced Abortion." New York and Washington DC: Alan Guttmacher Institute, *Facts in Brief,* January, 1997.
6. Gold, op. cit.
7. "Induced . . .," op. cit.
8. Ibid.
9. Ibid.
10. Ibid.
11. Ibid.
12. Ibid.
13. Cohen, Susan, and Rebecca Saul. "The Campaign Against Partial Birth Abortion: Status and Fallout." New York and Washington DC: Alan Guttmacher Institute, *The Guttmacher Report on Public Policy, Issues in Brief,* December, 1999, p. 6.
14. "Induced . . .," op. cit.
15. Ibid.
16. Ibid.
17. Ibid.
18. Ibid.
19. Gold, op. cit.
20. Induced . . .," op. cit.
21. "Mifepristone: Expanding Women's Options for Early Abortion." New York: Planned Parenthood Federation of America, *Fact Sheet,* December, 1999, pp. 1, 3.
22. "Induced . . .," op. cit.
23. Cohen, op. cit., p. 9.
24. "The Limitations of U.S. Statistics on Abortion." New York and Washington DC: Alan Guttmacher Institute, *Issues in Brief,* January, 1997.
25. "Partial Birth Abortion: What the Radical Right Doesn't Want You To Know." New York and Washington DC: National Council of Jewish Women, *Newsletter,* August, 1998.
26. "Teenagers' Right to Consent to Reproductive Health Care." New York and Washington DC: Alan Guttmacher Institute, *Issues in Brief,* October, 1997, p. 1.
27. "Parental Notification Act Faces Court Challenge in Colorado."

Washington DC: Advocates for Youth, *Advocate's Alert*, January, 1999.

28. "Bill Penalizing Abortion Aid Advances." Boston MA: *Boston Globe,* June 24, 1998, p. A19.

29. *Who Decides? A State-by-State Review of Abortion and Reproductive Rights, 1999.* Washington DC: National Abortion and Reproductive Rights Action League (NARAL), 1999, p. 8.

30. O'Hare, William P., editor. *Kids Count Data Book.* Baltimore MD: Annie E. Casey Foundation, 1999, p. 79.

31. Seelye, Katharine. "Congress Delays Voting on Budget Until Next Week." New York: *New York Times*, October 17, 1998, p. 1.

32. "Teenagers' Right to Consent . . .," op. cit.

33. Berger, Joseph. "Slain Physician Eulogized as Caring Man Who Defied Threats." New York: *New York Times*, October 27, 1998, p. A21.

34. Verhovek, Sam Howe. "Creators of Anti-Abortion Web Site Told to Pay Millions." New York: *New York Times*, February 3, 1999, p. A11.

35. Hernandez, Raymond. "Buffalo Clinic Vows to Continue Abortions." New York: *New York Times*, October 28, 1998, p. A23.

36. "Protection for Abortion Clinics." New York: *New York Times*, November 22, 1998, p. 16.

37. Gold, op. cit.

38. Cohen, op. cit.

39. Greenhouse, Linda. "Ex-Justice Blackmun Dies; Wrote Roe vs. Wade." Sarasota FL: *Sarasota Herald-Tribune*, March 5, 1999, p. 1.

Chapter 13. Attack Problems, Not People

1. Richards, David E. "Values and Sexual Health." New York and Washington DC: *SIECUS Report*, Vol. 18, #6, August/September, 1990.

2. Ketting, Evert. "Is the Dutch Abortion Rate Really That Low?" Utrecht, the Netherlands: NISSO, June, 1998.

3. Berne, Linda, and Barbara Huberman. *Aimer Sans Peur: European Approaches to Adolescent Sexual Behavior and Responsibility.* Washington DC: Advocates for Youth, 1999, pp. IX, XIII.

4. Ketting, op. cit.

5. Alford, Sue, and Ammie Feijoo. "Adolescent Sexual Health in Europe and the U.S. — Why the Difference?" Washington DC: Advocates for Youth, February, 2000.

6. Nosseo, Ilana. "Pregnancy and Childbearing Among Younger Teens." Washington DC: Advocates for Youth, *The Facts*, October, 1996.

7. Kirby, Douglas. *No Easy Answers: Research Findings on Programs to Reduce Teen Pregnancy*. Washington DC: National Campaign to Prevent Teen Pregnancy, March, 1997, p. 6.

8. Hayes, Michael, "Making Peace with Men: Building Bridges to Young Men and Fathers." New York: *PPFA Network*, Volume 3, #1, March, 2000, p. 1.

9. *Not Just for Girls: The Roles of Boys and Men in Teen Pregnancy Prevention*. Washington DC: National Campaign to Prevent Teen Pregnancy, November, 1997, p. 7.

10. "Teen Sex and Pregnancy." New York and Washington DC: Alan Guttmacher Institute, *Facts in Brief*, May, 1998.

11. Kirby, op. cit.

12. "Teenage Pregnancy: Developing Life Options." Arlington VA: American Association of School Administrators. New York: The Association of Junior Leagues, pp. 1-2.

13. *Sex and America's Teenagers*. New York and Washington DC: Alan Guttmacher Institute, 1994, p. 28.

14. "Teenage Pregnancy . . .," op. cit., pp. 3-4.

15. Maynard, Rebecca A., editor. *Kids Having Kids: Special Report on the Costs of Adolescent Childbearing*. New York: The Robin Hood Foundation Report, 1996, p. 19.

Chapter 14. You Can Help — Ten Points of Action

1. Fisher, Roger, and William Ury. *Getting to Yes*. New York: Penguin Books, 1983, pp. 41, 86, 154.

2. Burron, Arnold. "Traditionalist Christians and OBE: What's the Problem?" Alexandria VA: *Educational Leadership, March*, 1994, p. 73.

Books

Berne, Linda, and Barbara Huberman. *Aimer Sans Peur: European Approaches to Adolescent Sexual Behavior and Responsibility.* Washington DC: Advocates for Youth, 1999.

Brunner, Borgna, editor. *Time Almanac 2000 with Information Please.* Boston MA: Time, Inc., Home Entertainment, 1999.

Cohen, Mark Nathan. *The Culture of Intolerance.* New Haven: Yale University Press, 1998.

Daley, Daniel, and Vivian C. Wong. *Between the Lines.* New York: Fulton Press, 1999.

De Jong, William, and Jay A. Winsten. *The Media and the Message: Lessons Learned From Past Public Service Campaigns.* Washington DC: National Campaign to Prevent Teen Pregnancy, February, 1998.

Documenting the Power of Entertainment Television: The Impact of a Brief Health Message in One of TV's Most Popular Dramas. Menlo Park CA: Henry J. Kaiser Family Foundation, 1997.

Feijoo, Ammie N. *Teenage Pregnancy, The Case for Prevention.* Second Edition. Washington DC: Advocates for Youth, 1999.

Finer, Lawrence. *Evaluating Abstinence-Only Interventions.* Washington DC: National Campaign to Prevent Teen Pregnancy, 1998.

Fisher, Roger, and William Ury. *Getting to Yes.* New York: Penguin Books, 1983.

Gibb, Sarah, editor. *The Advocacy Manual for Sexuality Education, Health, and Justice: Resources for Communities of Faith.* Boston MA: Unitarian Universalist Association and United Church Board for Homeland Ministries, 1999.

Gold, Rachel Benson. *Abortion and Women's Health.* New York and Washington DC: Alan Guttmacher Institute, 1990.

Gore, Tipper. *Raising PG Kids in an X-Rated Society.* Nashville TN: Abingdon Press, 1987.

Guyer, Paul, editor. *Groundwork of the Metaphysics of Morality: Critical Essays.* New York: Roman and Littlefield, 1998.

Haffner, Debra W. *A Time to Speak: Faith Communities and Sexuality Education.* New York and Washington DC: Sex Information and Education Council of the United States (SIECUS), 1998.

Harris, Robie H. *It's Perfectly Normal: Changing Bodies, Growing Up, Sex and Sexual Health.* Cambridge MA: Candlewick Press, 1994.

Hatcher, Robert A., et al. *A Pocket Guide to Managing Contraception.* Tiger GA: Bridging the Gap Foundation, 1999.

Hunter, James D. *Culture Wars: The Struggle to Define America.* New York: Harper Collins, 1991.

Kirby, Douglas. *No Easy Answers: Research Findings on Programs to Reduce Teen Pregnancy.* Washington DC: National Campaign to Prevent Teen Pregnancy, March, 1997.

Lerman, Evelyn. *Teen Moms: The Pain and the Promise.* Buena Park CA: Morning Glory Press, 1997.

Loeb, Paul R. *Soul of a Citizen.* New York: St. Martin's Griffin Press, 1999.

Luker, Kristin. *Dubious Conceptions: The Politics of Teenage Pregnancy.* Cambridge MA: Harvard University Press, 1996.

Males, Mike A. *The Scapegoat Generation: America's War on Adolescents.* Monroe ME: Common Courage Press, 1996.

Maynard, Rebecca A., editor. *Kids Having Kids: Special Report on the Costs of Adolescent Childbearing.* New York: The Robin Hood Foundation Report, 1996.

Napier, Kristine. *The Power of Abstinence.* New York: Avon
 Books, 1996.

*Not Just for Girls: The Roles of Boys and Men in Teen Pregnancy
 Prevention.* Washington DC: National Campaign to Prevent Teen
 Pregnancy, November, 1997.

O'Hare, William P., editor. *Kids Count Data Book.* Baltimore MD:
 Annie E. Casey Foundation, 1999.

_____, editor. *When Teens Have Sex: Issues and Trends.* Baltimore
 MD: Annie E. Casey Foundation, 1998.

Pipher, Mary. *Reviving Ophelia.* New York: Ballantine Books, 1994.

Sartorius, Rolf. *Individual Conduct and Social Norms.* Encino CA:
 Dickinson, 1975.

Schurmann, Ann. *Baby Steps: Implementing Family Life Education in
 the Early Grades.* New Brunswick NJ: Network for Family Life
 Education, Rutgers, The State University of New Jersey, 1997.

_____. *No Accident: Adolescent Pregnancy in New Jersey Since
 1998.* New Brunswick NJ: Network for Family Life Education,
 Rutgers, The State University of New Jersey, 1998.

Sex and America's Teenagers. New York and Washington DC: Alan
 Guttmacher Institute, 1994.

Sher, George, editor. *Utilitarianism.* Indianapolis IN: Hackett
 Publishing Co., Inc., 1979.

Snapshots From the Front Line. Washington DC: National Campaign
 to Prevent Teen Pregnancy, May, 1997.

*While the Adults are Arguing, the Teens are Getting Pregnant: Over-
 coming Conflict in Teen Pregnancy Prevention.* Washington DC:
 National Campaign to Prevent Teen Pregnancy, August, 1998.

Whitehead, Barbara D., and Theodora Ooms. *Goodbye to Girlhood:
 What's Troubling Girls and What You Can Do About It.* Washington DC: National Campaign to Prevent Teen Pregnancy, 1999.

*Who Decides? A State-by-State Review of Abortion and Reproductive
 Rights, 1999.* Washington DC: National Abortion and Reproductive
 Rights Action League (NARAL), 1999.

Curricula

*Be Proud! Be Responsible! Strategies to Empower Youth to Reduce
 Their Risk for AIDS.* (Inner city youth, ages 13-18.) Select Media,
 1996. 1.800.343.5540.

Becoming a Responsible Teen. Santa Cruz CA: ETR Associates, 1997.
    1.800.321.4407.

Brick, Peggy, et al. *The New Teaching Safer Sex.* New Brunswick NJ:
    Center for Family Life Education, Planned Parenthood of Greater
    New Jersey, 1998. 973.539.9580, x120.

Brownlee, Patricia, et al. Video, "Considering Your Options."
    Washington DC: National Education Association Health
    Information Network, 1998. 1.800.229.4200.

Casparian, Elizabeth, Eva Goldfarb, Richard Kimball, Barbara Sprung,
    and Pamela M. Wilson. *Our Whole Lives: Comprehensive Sexuality
    Education.* Boston MA: Unitarian Universalist Association and
    United Church Board for Homeland Ministries, 1999.
    1.800.215.9076.

Focus on Kids: HIV Awareness. (Urban low income, ages 9-15.) Santa
    Cruz CA: ETR Associates, 1998. 1.800.321.4407.

Get Real About AIDS, Second Edition. Grades 9-12. Evanston IL:
    Altschul Group Corporation, 1988. 1.800.323.9084.

Girls Incorporated Preventing Adolescent Pregnancy. Indianapolis IN:
    National Resource Center. 317.634.7546.

Howard, Marion, and Marie Mitchell. *Postponing Sexual Involvement.*
    Atlanta GA: Adolescent Reproductive Health Center, Grady
    Hospital, 1995. 404.616.3513.

Life Management Skills. Sarasota FL: Sarasota Public Schools, 1998.
    941.486.2425.

*Reducing the Risk: Building Skills to Prevent Teen Pregnancy, STDs,
    and HIV.* (Grades 9, 10.) Santa Cruz CA: ETR Associates, 1996.
    1.800.321.4407.

Wasserman, Marie. *Learning About Family Life.* New Brunswick NJ:
    Network for Family Life Education, Rutgers, The State University
    of New Jersey, 1992. 732.445.7929.

Reports

"Abstinence Education Programs in Fiscal Year 1998." New York and
    Washington DC: Sex Information and Education Council of the
    United States (SIECUS), 1999.

Alford, Sue, and Ammie Feijoo. "Adolescent Sexual Health in Europe
    and the U.S. — Why the Difference?" Washington DC: Advocates
    for Youth, February, 2000.

Alford, Sue, and Gary Linnen, compilers. "Adolescents, HIV/AIDS and Other STDs." Washington DC: Advocates for Youth, November, 1998.

"ASHA Resource Guide: Facts to Think About." Research Triangle Park NC: American Social Health Association, August, 1995.

Berg, Eric. "Teens and HIV: Why Risk It?" Santa Cruz CA: ETR Associates, 1997.

Brindis, C., S. Paglano, and L. Davis. "Messengers and Methods for the New Millennium: A Round Table on Adolescents and Contraception." Washington, DC: Advocates for Youth Background Paper, February 10-11, 1999.

Brindis, Clarie D., et al. "Improving Adolescent Health: An Analysis and Synthesis of Health Policy Recommendations." San Francisco CA: National Adolescent Health Information Center, 1997.

Bumpus, Kristen. "Parent-Child Communication: Promoting Healthy Youth." Washington DC: Advocates for Youth, *The Facts,* February, 1999.

"Campaign Update." Washington DC: National Campaign to Prevent Teen Pregnancy, August/September 1996.

Clark, Peggy. "Awareness of Sexually Transmitted Diseases: An International Study." Research Triangle Park NC: American Social Health Association, August 27, 1995.

Cohen, Susan, and Rebecca Saul. "The Campaign Against Partial Birth Abortion: Status and Fallout." New York and Washington DC: Alan Guttmacher Institute, *The Guttmacher Report on Public Policy, Issues in Brief*, December, 1999.

"Confronting the Hidden Epidemic." Research Triangle Park NC: American Social Health Association, *Annual Report of ASHA.* 1996-97.

"Contraceptive Services." New York and Washington DC: Alan Guttmacher Institute, *Facts in Brief,* January, 1998.

Davis, Laura. "Adolescent Pregnancy and Childbearing." Washington DC: Advocates for Youth, *The Facts*, March, 1996.

_____. "Components of Promising Teen Pregnancy Prevention Programs." Washington DC: Advocates for Youth, *Issues at a Glance,* 1996.

"Equity in Prescription Insurance and Contraceptive Coverage Act of 1999." Washington DC: U.S. Congress, S.1200, February 22, 2000.

Flinn, Susan. "Abstinence-Until-Marriage Education: Unrealistic and Irresponsible." Washington DC: Advocates for Youth, *Issues at a*

Glance, February, 1998.

Folb, Kate. "A Report From the Media Project." Washington DC: Advocates for Youth, 1999.

"From Research to Classroom." Atlanta GA: Centers for Disease Control and Prevention, *Programs that Work.*

Gressle, Sharon. "Federal Civilian Employees and the FY 1999 Budget: CRS Issue Brief." Washington DC: Congressional Research Service, Library of Congress, October 30, 1998.

"Guidelines for Comprehensive Sexuality Education." New York and Washington DC: SIECUS *Fact Sheets*, March 18, 2000.

Haffner, Debra, and James Wagoner. "Vast Majority of Americans Support Sexuality Education." Washington DC: SIECUS, *SIECUS Report,* August/September, 1999.

Heilig, Steve. "Free Condoms in San Francisco Schools: Five Years and Running." San Francisco CA: San Francisco Medical Society, June 12, 1999.

Herdman, Cristina S. "Promising Adolescent Pregnancy Prevention Programs." Washington DC: Advocates for Youth, *Programs at a Glance,* 1996.

Hoffman, Anna. "Effective Comprehensive Sexuality Education." Washington DC: Advocates for Youth, *Programs at a Glance.* July, 1997.

Huston, Aletha, et al. "Measuring the Effects of Sexual Content in the Media." Menlo Park CA: Henry J. Kaiser Foundation, May, 1998.

"Induced Abortion." New York and Washington DC: Alan Guttmacher Institute, *Facts in Brief,* January, 1997.

"Into a New World: Young Women's Sexual and Reproductive Lives, Executive Summary." New York and Washington DC: Alan Guttmacher Institute, 1998.

Kearney, Sharon. "Title X Family Planning Program." Washington DC: Congressional Research Service of Congress, Library of Congress, *CRS Report*, October 26, 1998.

Kunkel, Dale, et al. "Sex on TV." Menlo Park CA: Kaiser Family Foundation, February, 1999.

Levenberg, Wrenn, compiler. "Adolescents and Abstinence." Washington DC: Advocates for Youth, *The Facts,* September, 1998.

"The Limitations of U.S. Statistics on Abortion." New York and Washington DC: Alan Guttmacher Institute, *Issues in Brief,* January, 1997.

MacNamara, Marina. "Adolescent Sexual Behavior: 1. Demographics."

Washington DC: Advocates for Youth, *The Facts,* 1997.

_____. "Adolescent Sexual Behavior: 2. Socio-Psychological Factors." Washington DC: Advocates for Youth, *The Facts,* July, 1997.

_____, compiler. "Adolescent Contraceptive Use." Washington DC: Advocates for Youth, *The Facts,* November, 1997.

_____, compiler. "Sexuality Education Curricula and Programs." Washington DC: Advocates for Youth, *The Facts,* September, 1997.

"Mifepristone: Expanding Women's Options for Early Abortion." New York: Planned Parenthood Federation of America, *Fact Sheet,* December, 1999.

Miller, Brent C. "A Research Synthesis of Family Influences on Adolescent Pregnancy." Washington DC: National Campaign to Prevent Teen Pregnancy, April, 1998.

Moore, Kristin A., et al. *The Child Indicator, #642.* Washington DC: Child Trends, 1999.

_____. *A Statistical Portrait of Adolescent Sex, Contraception, and Childbearing.* Washington DC: National Campaign to Prevent Teen Pregnancy, March, 1998.

"NC Poll: Most Voters Favor Condom Education." Research Triangle Park NC: American Social Health Association, May 28, 1996.

Norman, Jane, compiler. "Evaluated Peer Health Education Programs." Washington DC: Advocates for Youth, *Programs at a Glance,* November, 1999.

Nosseo, Ilana. "Pregnancy and Childbearing Among Younger Teens." Washington DC: Advocates for Youth, *The Facts,* October, 1996.

Ozer, E. M., and C. D. Brindis. "America's Adolescents: Are They Healthy?" San Francisco CA: Health Resources and Services Administration, University of California, San Francisco, 1998.

"Parental Notification Act Faces Court Challenge in Colorado." Washington DC: Advocates for Youth, *Advocate's Alert,* January, 1999.

"Partial Birth Abortion: What the Radical Right Doesn't Want You to Know." New York and Washington DC: National Council of Jewish Women, *Newsletter,* August, 1998.

"Postponing Sexual Involvement." Washington DC: Advocates for Youth, *Programs at a Glance,* July, 1997.

"Reproductive Health, Sex Education: Kansas Board Rejects Conservative Proposals." *Daily Health Reports,* November 6, 1998.

Rhodes, Chuck. "Health Risk Behavior Among Maine Youth." Atlanta GA: Centers for Disease Control, June, 1998.

Richards, David E. "Values and Sexual Health." New York and Washington DC: SIECUS, *SIECUS Report,* Vol. 18 #6, August/September, 1990.

Sadik, Nafis. "United Nations Population Fund Report." Washington DC: Advocates for Youth, November 16, 1998.

"Sex-Sensibility: Emergency Contraception Fact Sheet." Alexandria VA: American Medical Women's Association, November 17, 1999.

"Sexually Transmitted Disease in Maine." Augusta ME: Department of Human Services, *Annual Report,* 1997.

Solomon-Fears, Carmen. "Welfare Reform: Provisions Related to Non-marital Births." Washington DC: Congressional Research Service, Library of Congress, *CRS Report for Congress*, June 21, 1999.

STD News. Research Triangle Park NC: American Social Health Association, Spring/Summer, 1999.

"STD Q & A." Research Triangle Park NC: American Social Health Association, 1997.

Stevens, Jennifer, compiler. "Peer Education Promoting Healthy Behaviors." Washington DC: Advocates for Youth, *The Facts,* October, 1996.

"Teen Sex and Pregnancy." New York and Washington DC: Alan Guttmacher Institute, *Facts in Brief,* May, 1998.

"Teenage Pregnancy." Washington DC: Congressional Research Service, Library of Congress, *CRS Report for Congress,* October, 1999.

"Teenagers' Right to Consent to Reproductive Health Care." New York and Washington DC: Alan Guttmacher Institute, *Issues in Brief,* October, 1997.

"Tips for Teens." Washington DC: U.S. Department of Health and Human Services, Public Health Service Substance and Mental Health Administration.

"Trends in the HIV & AIDS Epidemic." Atlanta GA: Centers for Disease Control and Prevention, October 2, 1998.

Ventura, Stephanie J., et al. "Declines in Teenage Birth Rates: Update of National and State Trends." Hyattsville MD: Centers for Disease Control and Prevention, *National Vital Statistics Reports,* Vol. 47 #26, October 25, 1999.

"Victories and Vision, Equality, Equity, and Empowerment of Women." New York and Washington DC: National Council of Jewish Women, Vol. XI: Issue 8, April, 1999.

Wasem, Ruth E. "Abstinence Education Block Grant." Washington DC: Congressional Research Service, Library of Congress, *CRS Report for Congress*, September 15, 1997.

Witte, Kim. "Scare Tactics Promote Improved Behavior Only With Right Combination." Silver Springs MD: CD Publications, *AIDS/ HIV Surveillance Report,* Volume 11, #1, September 23, 1998.

Articles

"Appraising Teen Magazines." New Brunswick NJ: *Family Life Matters*. Network for Family Life Education, Rutgers, the State University of New Jersey, Spring, 1998.

Berger, Joseph. "Slain Physician Eulogized as Caring Man Who Defied Threats." New York: *New York Times,* October 27, 1998.

"Bill Penalizing Abortion Aid Advances." Boston MA*: Boston Globe,* June 24, 1998.

Blum, Robert, and Peggy M. Rinehart. "Protecting Adolescents from Harm: Findings from the National Longitudinal Study of Adolescent Health." *Journal of the American Medical Association (JAMA),* September, 1997.

Brody, Jane E. "Teenagers and Sex: Younger and More at Risk." New York: *New York Times,* September 15, 1998.

Brown, L., and R. DiClemente. "Predictors of Condom Use in Sexually Active Adolescents." Palo Alto CA: *Journal of Adolescent Health,* Vol. 13, 1992.

Burges, Don. "Archdeacon Calls for Condoms in the Schools." Hamilton Bermuda: *Bermuda Sun,* February 7,1996.

Burron, Arnold. "Traditionalist Christians and OBE: What's the Problem?" Alexandria VA: *Educational Leadership,* March, 1994.

"Church Convicts Pastor for Blessing Gay Union." Sarasota FL: *Sarasota Herald-Tribune*, Sept. 9, 1999.

Clarity, James F. "Scandals and New Beliefs Changing Ireland's Church." New York: *New York Times,* June 13, 1999.

"Click Here for the 21st Century Learning." Cambridge MA: *Harvard Graduate School of Education Bulletin*, Winter/Spring, 1999.

"Condom Availability for Youth." Elk Grove IL: *Journal of the American Academy of Pediatrics*, Vol. 95 #2, February, 1995.

"Contraception, Three Days After." New York: *New York Times*, September 4, 1998.

Delbanco, Suzanne F., et al. "Are We Making Progress with Emergency Contraception?" Alexandria VA: *Journal of American Medical Women's Association,* Volume 53, #5, November 17, 1999.

DiClemente, R., M. Durbin, et al. "Determinants of Condom Use Among Junior High School Students in a Minority Inner-City District." Elk Grove IL: *Journal of American Pediatrics,* Vol. 89, 1992.

Dillon, Sam. "Smaller Families to Bring Big Change in Mexico." New York: *New York Times,* June 8, 1999.

Ellertson, Charlotte, et al. "Should Emergency Contraceptive Pills Be Available Without Prescription?" Alexandria VA: *Journal of American Medical Women's Association,* Volume 53, #5, November 17, 1999.

Freedman, Alix M. "Why Teenage Girls Love 'The Shot'; Why Others Aren't So Sure." New York: *Wall Street Journal,* October 14, 1998.

Greenhouse, Linda. "Ex-Justice Blackmun Dies; Wrote Roe vs. Wade." Sarasota FL: *Sarasota Herald-Tribune,* March 5, 1999.

Handelman, Jay. "Let's Talk About Sex and Cancer." Sarasota FL: *Sarasota Herald-Tribune,* September 22, 1998.

Hayes, Michael. "Making Peace with Men: Building Bridges to Young Men and Fathers." New York: *PPFA Network,* Volume 3, #1, March, 2000.

Henshaw, Stanley K. "Abortion Incidence and Services in the U.S. 1995-1996." New York and Washington DC: Alan Guttmacher Institute, *Family Planning Perspectives,* Volume 30, #6, November/December, 1998.

Hernandez, Raymond. "Buffalo Clinic Vows to Continue Abortions." New York: *New York Times,* October 28, 1998.

Hollingsworth, Catherine. "South Is an Example of the Changing Face of AIDS." Sarasota FL: *Sarasota Herald-Tribune,* February 2, 1998.

Hollins, Mark. "Pill Bill Critics Say Insurance Would Suffer." Sarasota FL: *Sarasota Herald-Tribune,* March 12, 1999.

Holmes, Steven A. "Right to Abortion Quietly Advances in State Courts." New York: *New York Times,* December 6, 1998.

"Huge Gains and Huge Worries on AIDS." New York: *New York Times,* October 9, 1998.

Ibrahim, Youssef M. "Aids Is Slashing Africa's Population." New York: *New York Times,* October 28, 1998.

Jamieson, Kathleen Hall. ". . . and Now for Some Good News." Washington DC: *AARP News,* October, 1998.

Kegeles, S., N. Adler, and C. Irwin. "Adolescents and Condoms: The Association of Beliefs with Intentions to Use." *American Journal of Diseases of Children* 143:911-915, 1989.

Ketting, Evert. "Is the Dutch Abortion Rate Really that Low?" Utrecht, the Netherlands: Netherlands Institute for Social Sexological Research, June, 1998.

Maganini, Steven, Andy Furillo, and Ralph Montano. "Three Synagogues Struck by Arson." Sacramento CA: *Sacramento Bee*, June 19, 1999.

"Male Myths Leave Guys Worried." New Brunswick NJ: *Sex Etc, a Newsletter for Teens by Teens*. Winter, 1999.

Niebuhr, Gustav. "Methodist Leaders Must Weigh Penalties." New York: *New York Times*, June 11, 1999.

"Protection for Abortion Clinics." New York: *New York Times,* November 22, 1998.

Richardson, Lynda. "School Data Show Free Condoms Don't Affect Sex Rates." New Brunswick NJ: *Daily News*, Campaign for Children, October 2, 1997.

Rickman, R. L., and M. Lodico. "Sexual Communication Is Associated with Condom Use by Sexually Active Incarcerated Adolescents." Palo Alto CA: *Journal of Adolescent Health,* Vol. 13, 1994.

Rimel, Rebecca W. "A Power to Motivate or Manipulate." New York: *New York Times*, February 14, 1999.

Rodriguez, Monica, Rebecca Young, Stacie Renfro, Marysol Asencio, and Debra Haffner."Teaching Our Teachers to Teach, A SIECUS Study on Training and Preparation for HIV/AIDS Prevention and Sexuality Education." New York and Washington DC: SIECUS, December 1995/January 1996.

Rodriguez, Pablo. "The Doctor Is in the Bulletproof Vest." New York: *New York Times*, October 28, 1998.

Rosin, Hanna. "Rabbi Group Sanctions Gay Unions." Sarasota FL: *Sarasota Herald-Tribune,* March 30, 2000.

Saewyc, Elizabeth M., Linda H. Bearinger, Robert W. Blum and Michael D. Resnick. "Sexual Intercourse, Abuse and Pregnancy Among Adolescent Women: Does Sexual Orientation Make a Difference?" New York: Alan Guttmacher Institute, *Family Planning Perspectives,* Volume 31, Number 3, May/June 1999.

"School Condom Availability and Condom Use Among Teens." Washington DC: Advocates for Youth, *Transitions,* Vol. 10 #1. September 9, 1998.

Seelye, Katharine. "Congress Delays Voting on Budget Until Next

Week." New York: *New York Times*, October 17, 1998.

Sterngold, James. "Lessons Not Quite Ready for Prime Time." New York: *New York Times*, March 28, 1999.

"Teen Thoughts on Condom Distribution." New Brunswick NJ: *Daily News,* Campaign for Children, August 29, 1997.

Torres, Aida, and Jacqueline D. Forrest. "Why Do Women Have Abortions?" New York: Alan Guttmacher Institute, *Family Planning Perspectives,* Vol. 120, #4, July/August, 1998.

Trussell, Dr. James. "Emergency Contraception: It Can Change Our World." New Brunswick, NJ: *Family Life Matters*, #36, Winter 1999.

Verhovek, Sam Howe. "Creators of Anti-Abortion Web Site Told to Pay Millions." New York: *New York Times*, February 3, 1999.

"Who We Are." New Brunswick NJ: Network for Family Life Education, Rutgers, The State University of New Jersey, www.sxetc.org, February, 1999.

Booklets/Miscellaneous

"HIV/AIDS Prevention Workshop for Teens." Palo Alto CA: Aids Prevention Program, YWCA Flyer.

Johnson-Green, Sharon. "Ten Good Reasons Not to Be a Teenage Parent." Santa Cruz CA: Journeyworks Publishing; Johnson City TN: Center for Women's Health.

"Loving Safely: What You Need to Know About STDs." Research Triangle Park NC: American Social Health Association, 1998.

"Nine Tips to Help Faith Leaders and Their Communities Address Teen Pregnancy." Washington DC: National Campaign to Prevent Teen Pregnancy, November, 1998.

Rinehart, Peggy M. "Connections that Make a Difference in the Lives of Youth." Washington DC: National Campaign to Prevent Teen Pregnancy, 1998.

"Sexually Transmitted Diseases (STDs): What You Need to Know." Research Triangle Park NC: American Social Health Association, 1997.

"Teenage Pregnancy: Developing Life Options." Arlington, VA: American Association of School Administrators; New York: The Association of Junior Leagues.

"Ten Tips for Parents to Help Their Children Avoid Teen Pregnancy." Washington DC: National Campaign to Prevent Teen Pregnancy, 1998.

INDEX

About the Author

Evelyn Lerman, the youngest of three daughters, was raised in a strong woman's world. Everyone had an opinion and everyone wanted to be right. Very early on she decided her role was to listen, not take sides, and try to find a reasonable, practical solution.

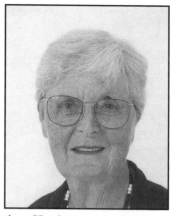

She took this attitude with her into her careers of parenting, teaching, camp directing, and mediating. Her interest in people led her to interviewing and writing for newspapers in high school and majoring in journalism in college. While there, she worked on the newspaper and the yearbook. After graduation she married and became the writer, editor, and everything-in-chief of the family business trade journal for ten years. During her teaching career she authored innumerable curriculum units and contributed to a book on writing. She has graduate degrees in education and in human development.

She is the author of ***Teen Moms: The Pain and the Promise*** (1997), a book about the realities of life as a teen mother. Teen mothers shared their stories which Lerman expertly combined with the research showing 80-85 percent of teen mothers are poor, the majority were sexually abused as children, and most of the fathers of their babies are older than they are. Many of the youngest mothers were impregnated by adult men. ***Teen Moms*** shows clearly that teen pregnancy prevention is not as simple as insisting that "Those girls should just say 'No'."

Safer Sex: The New Morality outlines the changes our culture must make to help our youth avoid too-early pregnancy, sexually transmitted infections, and the need for abortions.

Retired from her work with the schools, Lerman still teaches writing to adults and directs a reading program for teen mothers. She and Allie, who have been married for 52 years, have two children and four grandchildren.